GOD'S KEY TO HEALTH AND HAPPINESS

GOD'S KEY TO HEALTH AND HAPPINESS

ELMER A. JOSEPHSON

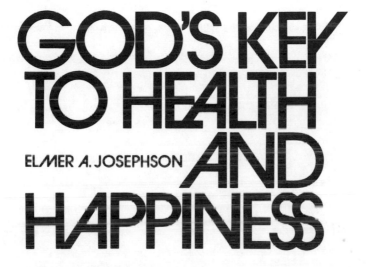

Fleming H. Revell Company
Old Tappan, New Jersey

Scripture quotations in this volume are based on the King James Version of the Bible.

ISBN-0-8007-5018-7

TO the Lord of Life, the One God of Abraham, Isaac and Jacob, the Covenant God of Israel, the Messiah, Redeemer of His people and His quickening Spirit, Who "giveth wisdom, out of whose mouth cometh knowledge and understanding," be all glory and praise forever, and ever.

Contents

7

Acknowledgments

To my good wife who worked untiringly, offering helpful suggestions, making corrections, typing many drafts of the entire manuscript, whose cheerful spirit and constant encouragement have been of inestimable help and blessing.

To Dr. Thomas H. Nelson, former president of the American Bible School, editor of the *Ram's Horn;* Dr. Hall, late chief of the Division of Zoology of the U.S. Public Health Service; Senator Thomas C. Desmond, chairman of the New York Trichinosis Commission; Dr. Hess and Dr. Clark of Ashland, Ohio; Dr. Paul Dudley White, President Eisenhower's heart doctor; Dr. William Brady, physician-surgeon and news columnist; Sir Edward Mellanby, British research scientist; and Catharyn Elwood, author of *Feel Like a Million,* Devin-Adair Publishers, New York, our deep appreciation.

To *Reader's Digest* for their special written permission to publish excerpts from an article written by Dr. Laird S. Goldsborough, and to Sir James Paget of London, England.

Our deep appreciation to Eleanor Baerg, our office secretary who had the mammoth task of 'composing' the type of the entire volume, and to other secretaries and assistants who contributed much in typing drafts and checking manuscripts, and to other members of our staff that assisted in many ways.

To many contributors and friends for their helpful information and my apologies to many others we have failed to mention and to some who prefer to remain anonymous, our thanks.

INTRODUCTION
One Thing We All Want and Need

What is the first interest of adults around the world? Is it love, romance, sex, money, success, popularity, fame? No. All of these would run a very poor second, and without 'the first,' most of these would hold little value. All other earthly blessings and joys lose their charm and attraction without it.

The University of Chicago, The American Association of Adult Education, and The United Y.M.C.A. Schools, made a survey that covered two years and cost many thousands of dollars in order to answer this question. The survey revealed that the first interest of people everywhere is *health*. Nothing can be fully enjoyed, most things can never be attained without it.

This being the case, everyone should be interested in the contents of this book. But let me warn you—only those with an open mind should read it. The truths set forth here are revolutionary. They run counter to public opinion. They cut across years of commonly accepted eating customs, and uproot deeply embedded dietary habits. But don't put up a guard. This book, by the grace of God, could awaken you to a new life of health and happiness. But. . . .

II

Happiness

What is happiness? Isn't it getting your heart's greatest desire? Solomon wrote, "Hope deferred maketh the heart sick: but when the desire cometh, it is a tree of life" (Proverbs 13:12). However, if our desires are wrong, their fulfillment will only mock us.

Our supreme desire depends upon our situation. Happiness to a man with a severe stomach ailment would be to enjoy his meals again. Happiness to a man dying with cancer would be deliverance from the dreaded disease. To a man sentenced to life imprisonment, freedom would be his chief desire, and to a man under sentence of death, the promise of life would be the sweetest word he could hear. This is the wonderful hope that the Book of God holds out to every man.

Man, with much study, effort, expense and daring, has broken the space barrier, not to mention the various others. We are launching rockets and satellites at enormous expense, to see what may be learned from the heavens. Isn't it time we break through the 'poor-nutrition barrier,' and come through with the good sound health that the Almighty intended for us to enjoy?

Shall we surrender because of the barriers and obstacles that the critical prophets of gloom, discouragement, ridicule and unbelief throw in the way? Nehemiah met them in 445 BC, but they did not deter him. Their laughs, jeers, scorning and opposition only accelerated the work. He went on with the building of the wall . . . and finished it . . . and so shall we, by the grace of God.

For the Open-Minded

Don't throw this book down and reject its truths because of its new concepts: you may detour around your own health and future happiness. And do not let prejudice, which has plagued us all, rob you of these riches. So many times we hold prejudices to our own hurt. But remember, a bed of languishing illness and incurable disease can be so hard and long, and death is so final. "Remember now thy Creator [and His Word] . . . before the evil days [sickness and suffering as the chapter indicates] come, when thou shalt say, I have no pleasure in them" (Ecclesiastes 12:1). I earnestly pray your life will be enriched by the truths revealed in these pages. If you invest the time, you will reap the dividends.

This is not a literary treatise or a critical analysis on the subject of health. Technical language has purposely been avoided. Although these truths are scientific as well as Biblical, we have tried to write in laymen's language so that the "man on the street" can understand. My great concern is the health and future welfare of this and succeeding generations to the glory of the all-wise Creator.

This book is not for the person with a closed mind. Those who refuse to grow never develop—they soon die. How can anyone who knows all, learn any more? He sits as a judge over all the earth. "Fools despise wisdom and instruction" (Proverbs 1:7).

One of the saddest things one can experience is to meet a seemingly promising young man or young lady with winning ways and natural ability but who refuses instruction. I have tried to kindly counsel such, that they might avoid heartaches, pitfalls, disease or even possible imprisonment and premature death. How tragic and self-destructive to hear them retort, "Don't lecture me." The Scriptures declare such are fools that are headed for the quicksand and they will eat the bread of affliction.

Success

On the other hand, what a refreshing, joyful experience it is to speak to those who are wise and ready to hear instruction. Our God declares of them, "A wise man will hear and will increase learning; and a man of understanding shall attain unto wise counsels" (Proverbs 1:5). For "His delight is in the law of the Lord; and in His law doth he meditate day and night. And he shall be like a tree planted by the rivers of water, that bringeth forth his fruit in his season; his leaf also shall not wither; and whatsoever he doeth shall prosper" (Psalm 1:2,3).

"This book of the law shall not depart out of thy mouth; but thou shalt meditate therein day and night, that thou mayest observe to do according to all that is written therein: for then thou shalt make thy way prosperous, and then thou shalt have good success" (Joshua 1:8).

GOD'S KEY TO HEALTH AND HAPPINESS

1

Why the Book Was Written

The Cause

"Of making many books there is no end. . . ." Solomon was right, but this is not just another book but a revolutionary war —war against sickness and misery, aches and pains, against a subtle killer—war against satanic forces that hate the truth that makes us free. I am anxious to put in your hands, reader, the weapon of victory, the truths that have restored and prolonged my life and added much true happiness.

"Is there not a cause?" David answered his brothers when they accused him of coming down merely to see the battle between Israel and the Philistines. They charged him with being completely out of character and insisted that he should be back in the wilderness tending his father's sheep. But the Hebrew nation was being oppressed and about to come under the heel of a cruel and ruthless enemy. David's heart was on fire for Israel's deliverance and he knew he had the answer. He pressed his claims even against his own family's objections and disapproval but he won a great victory.

In this matter, also, there is a great cause at stake. Many are losing the battle for health and even for life itself. Why? Let the *Lord* answer, "My people are destroyed for lack of knowledge" . . . and with many, "because thou hast rejected knowledge"

(Hosea 4:6). This is true physically as well as spiritually.

David lamented after Abner had been slain by Joab, "Died Abner as a fool dieth?" (II Samuel 3:27–39). His life was safe and guaranteed to him inside the walls of the city of refuge. Joab asked to speak to him outside the gate and he foolishly stepped outside of the area of his safety to death.

If David had known of Joab's plot, he would have tried desperately to get a message of warning to Abner in order to save his life, but Joab hid it from David. Many today are not aware of a subtle enemy who would induce them to step outside the safety zone of God's Word, to disease and an untimely death. Is not this suffering and dying like a fool?

The Knowledge

I, too, am desperately concerned about getting a message through to my generation, and to you, reader, that you may come to a knowledge of this truth which I am convinced can deliver the sick and dying. I speak with no uncertainty, for it raised me almost literally out of the grave.

This book is written at the suggestion and insistence of many trusted friends, as well as from my own earnest desire to make this truth of deliverance known. This is a debt that I owe first to God, for graciously revealing this blessed truth, and secondly to my fellow men that they may be set free, not only from sickness and disease, but from its very fear which in itself is a destroyer.

In the olden days before the network of hard surface highways, there was always the fear of getting stuck in the mud when starting out on cross-country driving. When dark clouds came up, they were the cause of real concern and worry. Many did get hopelessly bogged down, which delayed them hours and even days. What a relief it was when someone could direct you to a paved road that would guarantee a mud-free trip all the way to your destination.

God's laws are paved highways that keep us from getting bogged down in all sorts of miseries and needless difficulties. To know we are travelling on them relieves us of the fears that plague the future of so many today and assures us of a safe and on-schedule arrival. Happy is the man who gets off the mud road of his own prejudice and preconceived concepts, on to the paved highway, the Word of the Almighty, "whose ways are perfect."

The Application

God has given directions for the care of the *body,* which is His temple and habitation, as well as for the *spirit* and we shall give an account to Him for both. We have been made the custodians of God's house, the dwelling place of His Spirit's presence. We are to count it a sacred trust that, as Christian believers, we may have a good report at the judgment seat of Jesus Christ.

Vital organs and members of the body must first be destroyed before the body itself succumbs. And so it can be said that heart, lungs, bowels, kidneys, liver, etc., are destroyed because the person lacked knowledge or rejected knowledge. Many die because they have no knowledge of preventive measures; others perish of various diseases because they do not know of the remedy. A tragedy seems so much greater if the victim has been warned of impending death and disregards a proven cure. "Because thou hast rejected knowledge, I also will reject thee," the Lord declares.

The heart-rending thing about most tragedies is that they cannot be undone, and some diseases gain such headway they cannot be stopped. In the light of this sober fact, earnestly consider the truths in the following chapters.

There is not the slightest doubt in my mind that I would have been in my grave years ago had I not come to a knowledge of this key to health and happiness. I know of many who have died who, as the Lord said through Hosea, "are destroyed for lack of knowledge." If through the testimony and evidence presented here I can save some (I trust there will be countless numbers) from an untimely death that their mouths may continue longer to praise our matchless Redeemer and show forth His deliverance, then the years of study and research, time, suffering and cost will be well worth it all.

Apart from the Holy Scriptures, I suppose there is no book written that you and I agree with fully. (But, reader, if you doubt *Holy Writ,* this volume will hold little for you, since it is based on the Eternal Word.) It is so natural for us to have deep prejudices that are not easily erased. We may heatedly contend that these are strong convictions on our part; however, in a transparent examination of our beliefs in the light of eternal truth, we many times find them colored with dark conclusions of bias and prejudice. These preconceived concepts and dyed-in-the-wool "I'm right; I won't change" ideas, often blind us and close our minds to new truths that would transform our stagnant lives into fountains of blessing and our wilderness into gardens of Eden. May our Lord give us cool eyes and His guiding Spirit of truth to lead us into a knowledge of the whole counsel of God.

Since the Creator of the universe needs no letters of recommendation from us, or any supporting data to back His claims, therefore, the scientific information, the facts, the figures and other such findings from great universities are included in the book merely as illustrations and explanations, not as proof or evidence.

In the book of Job, after all the wide discussion of tragedies and joys of life by those who were considered the wise men of that day, we read, "The Lord answered Job out of the whirlwind, Where were you when I laid the foundations of the earth? Who laid the cornerstone . . . who shut up the sea with doors [when He said, "Hitherto shalt thou come but no further and here shall thy proud waves be stayed."] . . . who provides food for the raven," etc.? In chapters 38 through 41, scores of questions are asked that man cannot answer. In chapter 42 Job comes to the conclusion that God is the maker and doer of all things . . . "That they may know from the rising of the sun and from the west that there is none beside me, I am the Lord and there is none else" (Isaiah 45:6).

Another important introductory word: *This is one volume that must be read carefully from the beginning to end, in order to get the undistorted picture.* Do not draw conclusions at the close of any one paragraph or chapter. Please do not play leap frog or take a passage out of its context which does not do justice to yourself or to the book. Read it in its entirety before drawing a final conclusion.

NOTE: We will repeat certain principles and facts throughout the book that we feel are essential to the immediate subject matter. This is not "vain repetition." This is done deliberately to drive home the importance of these various truths in their different relationships.

Some have written asking if the author is still living. Yes, very much so and I am in most excellent health, feeling like a "kid," due to the applied truths found in this volume and, of course, by God's grace and sovereign watchcare.

I sincerely pray that the Spirit of God will make this book a blessing to you, and I humbly and reverently add, "Blessed is he that readeth."

2

The Foundation

Writer's Credentials

How could I live with my conscience and answer to God? How can I keep silent when many of my friends are dropping on beds of sickness and disease and even into their graves from the same causes that brought me into the very jaws of death about forty years ago? I found this wonderful truth of deliverance in the pages of the Book of God. Why didn't I write it sooner? First, people do not readily accept advice such as this, of a young man. Secondly, I wanted to be "doubly sure" and fully prove this truth over a period of years, which I have done now since 1936.

My credentials are the forty years that I have used the "tools" that God put in my hands. The laboratory in which these tools and instruments were tested is my body, which today is a memorial to this applied Biblical and scientific truth.

I was plagued with many things such as gall bladder trouble, running piles, kidney disorder, arthritis, etc.; but the mental suffering from a nervous breakdown was far greater than even these physical ailments.

In the summer of 1936, after my complete nervous breakdown, a doctor, who knew my case, turned to me and said as casually as he would talk about the weather, "They are going to be playing the slow music after you before long." He stated that I had a carcinoma (cancer) of the stomach. There were periods of seven to ten days at a time that I could not even keep water down but vomited it up green. It seemed I would literally starve to death.

I had tried everything . . . home remedies, patent medicines, costly prescriptions, various doctors and was prayed for by those who believed in divine healing. I continued losing ground and dropped in weight from 155 pounds to 115 pounds. I finally planned my own funeral service and believed that 1936 or 1937 would be inscribed on my grave-marker. One instance during this time stands out clearly in my mind. I was visiting the home of my sister, Mrs. Evelyn Philgreen. My nephew, Irving, her first-born, then 18 months old was toddling in the yard outside. I thought to myself, "I will never live to see him graduate from any school, much less come to adulthood. I am doomed to death." But out of the abyss of this darkness, I began to see the light breaking through the Scriptures, which brought wonderful healing and deliverance to me. It is this shining truth I wish to pass on to you.

Hezekiah turned his face to the wall and prayed, and God added to him 15 years. I turned my heart to the Word of God and obeyed, and since that time, He has added unto me 40 years. Not only did I see a lovely niece and twin nephews born, but I saw Irving graduate from high school and university, marry, have children, and enter the ministry. I can testify with the Psalmist, "He sent His Word and healed me" (Psalm 107:20). How wonderful are His words, "For they are life unto those who find them, and health to all their flesh" (Proverbs 4:22).

Are you sick and bound by some ailment or disease? Can you believe that there is real genuine and lasting health available to you? I believe it with all my heart. It is the promise of God who cannot lie.

The Crux of the Matter

As a young minister I had only sympathy for those who spoke seriously of "diet." "Diet" was often the butt of my jokes. Diet to me meant cutting out everything you enjoyed eating just for the sake of becoming stylishly thin or because one was sick and ready for the undertaker. I ridiculed special nutrition since I honestly believed that you could eat anything you wished and God would keep you well. "After all," I reasoned, "isn't He God? Isn't He greater than all and doesn't He have all power?" And so I foolishly gloried in the fact that I had greater faith than all those who were sick and had to be so careful as to what they ate.

It was this sort of thinking that all but destroyed me. I had failed to take into account that God had set up the universe on a foundation of laws that govern all of life on every plane, in every sphere and at every level. Here I was brought up short and made to realize something of the truth, "To the law and to the testimony: if they speak not according to this word, it is because there is no light in them" (Isaiah 8:20).

I read recently of a supposedly very intelligent man who said he was so busy he had no time to think about what he ate. Let's hope he did not make the statement merely to impress people. He would not say regarding building a house that he was so busy he had no time to think of the materials that went into it. It is far more important to check the "building blocks" that go into the construction of the organic house of our bodies than that which goes into the making of inorganic houses of wood and stone. If we do not, it will come tumbling down much sooner than the Chief Architect planned. The law of "cause and effect" is operative in both.

A B Cs of Diet

God *could* keep you *alive* supernaturally without your eating food, but He doesn't do it—It is not His plan. God *could* keep you *well* supernaturally without your eating right, but He *does not*—It is not His plan. This law, as implied by Jesus in Matthew 4:4, states that you must have bread and food in order to exist—live physically.

A dear godly pastor in southern Missouri, desperately seeking for a spiritual awakening in his church, fasted beyond the point of no return (several weeks) and died as a result. He was seeking a spiritual blessing but broke a physical law and so forfeited his life.

Settle this truth—As it is *not* in God's plan to keep you *alive without eating,* so it is *not* in God's plan to keep you *well without eating right!* If you do not eat food you will die; if you do not eat good food you will not have good health. If you eat bad food you will have bad health. No food = no life. Bad food = bad health. Good food = good health. Live foods = live bodies. Dead foods = dead bodies. — It is as simple as that.

Reading this book will not be a wild goose chase or a case of just "huntin' goat feathers." The time spent will pay lasting dividends. You may not find gold at the end of this rainbow, but you will find something far better—a solid foundation upon which to build a well and strong body. My thanksgiving goes unto the Lord of Life, Who opened my mind and His Word to me. Most of these truths are rooted in Holy Scriptures, are verified by modern science and have been tested through over forty years of experience. These are my credentials.

You will find no grinding of a commercial axe, no selling of synthetic pills or capsules, no peddling of claptrap gadgets or difficult exercises to go through. It is merely a down-to-earth common sense and exhilarating way of life and health.

One well-to-do Texas rancher, who had suffered for years with a "bad stomach," after observing these truths for one year said, "Elmer, you have saved me over $1,000." (He felt so good he bought his pastor [not me] a new automobile.)

You will not only gain knowledge gathered from over forty years of research, and reap the benefits from that many years' experience and of lessons learned through much physical affliction and suffering that was conquered by these truths, *but* you can also become the grateful possessor of sound, vibrant health, and thereby add many years of usefulness and happiness to your own life. God grant it.

3

As a Man Thinketh

The Power of "Seed Thought"

The potential power of the human mind is beyond the "probe-ability" of man to fully comprehend. Man has experimented and experienced enough to learn this. We do know, however, before a man can accomplish anything, there must first be the seed-thought planted in the mind. The idea, the plan or undertaking must be nourished, developed and deeply rooted in the mind. You must be "sold on it."

You must settle every move before you make it in this intricate and precision equipment that Solomon refers to as the "heart." He wrote: "As a man thinketh in his heart, so is he" (Proverbs 23:7). And, "Keep thy heart with all diligence; for out of it are the issues of life" (Proverbs 4:23).

God has committed unto man and made him the responsible trustee of this powerful instrument. It can blight or bless us according to our use of it.

"Positive Thinking" According To The Scriptures

Volumes have been written by many writers on "positive thinking." The Apostle Paul also believed in it and the Spirit of God inspired it, as recorded in Philippians 4:8. He lists various positive virtues and declares, "Whatsoever things are true, whatsoever things are honest, whatsoever things are just, whatsoever things are pure, whatsoever things are lovely, whatsoever things are of good report; if there be any virtue, and if there be any praise, think on these things." Thoughts are the seeds from which the plant of action grows, and this growth is governed by law.

First, then, in regard to your own health, you must be fully convinced in your mind that it is God's will for you to be well, according to the Word of God. If you are not convinced of this, your mind will yield to sickness and to satanic forces and you cannot be delivered. We who believe the Bible to be the infallible Word of God must find our answers there. What saith the Scriptures? Does God promise health and long life, everything being equal? Let us consider these promises and may they take deep root in our hearts.

"My son, forget not my law; but let thine heart keep my commandments: for length of days, and long life, and peace, shall they add to thee" (Proverbs 3:1,2).

"Be not wise in thine own eyes: fear the Lord, and depart from evil. It shall be health to thy navel, and marrow to thy bones" (Proverbs 3:7,8).

"Hear, O my son, and receive my sayings; and the years of thy life shall be many" (Proverbs 4:10).

"My son, attend to my words; incline thine ear unto my sayings. Let them not depart from thine eyes; keep them in the midst of thine heart. For they are life unto those that find them, and health to all their flesh" (Proverbs 4:20–22).

In the New Testament we find Jesus "healed all that were sick" (Matthew 8:16). ". . . healing every sickness and every disease among the people" (Matthew 9:35).

As you follow the ministry of the Lord through the gospels, you will find His will totally expressed to the leper who came and worshipped Him saying, "Lord, if thou wilt, thou canst make me clean." Jesus said, "I will, be thou clean," and his leprosy was cleansed (Matthew 8:2,3).

"Exceptions to Healing"

You may say, "But there are exceptions!" Yes, God does use sickness:

(1) for testing, as in the case of Job;

(2) in disciplinary measures, as Paul declared in Hebrews 12;

(3) for judgments—I Corinthians 11:29,30.

But if we are convinced the sickness is God's discipline, then, should we see a doctor and seek recovery through other medicinal means? Let us not pull away from the corrective lash. If a disease is divine chastening, it generally will be cured only as the individual confesses his sin and begins a new obedience unto God.

Heart Attitude a Key

God gave Solomon wisdom above all men as the Scriptures relate, "He was wiser than all men." We should, therefore, take his advice. Solomon admonishes, "Keep thy heart with all diligence, for out of it are the issues of life" (Proverbs 4:23). The "heart," or mind, is the seat of our moral emotions and affections and responsible choices. Our loves shape our lives. Solomon warns, keep these under control. "A sound heart is the life of the flesh, but envy the rottenness of the bones" (Proverbs 14:30).

"By sorrow of the heart, the spirit is broken" (Proverbs 15:13).

"A merry heart doeth good like a medicine: but a broken spirit drieth the bones" (Proverbs 17:22).

"The spirit of a man will sustain his infirmity, but a wounded spirit who can bear?" (Proverbs 18:14).

Right attitudes encourage and refresh the soul and strengthen the moral spirit; actually, then the blood and the sympathetic nervous system are rejuvenated, which make for good cell construction and builds healthy body tissues.

Wrong relationships and attitudes depress the mind and fill the blood with an alkaloid poison. The involuntary sympathetic nerve system actually causes a malformation of cell construction and tissue arrangement.

Under chemical analysis, every secretion in the body of a cheerful and contented person is found to be largely free of destructive toxins. However, the same chemical test taken of those who harbor hate, envy, anger, fear and jealousy, or who are beset by fear, worry and anxiety, are found to produce toxins in the blood that are destructive to one's physical welfare.

In III John 2 the Apostle John, inspired by God's Spirit, writes, "Beloved, I wish above all things that thou mayest prosper and be in health, even as thy soul prospereth." *So settle this:* It is God's will for you to be well and to enjoy life and health.

Sometimes we may be "perplexed, but not in despair" (II Corinthians 4:8) as to God's will for us, whether we should go or stay, whether to be here or there, in this ministry or that, etc. But how wonderful when God's will is so clearly indicated, as it is in this and other passages, i.e., it is our Lord's desire for us to be strong physically as well as spiritually.

We will not deal here with the subject of divine healing or miracles which, without question, are taught both in the so-called 'Old' and in the New Testaments. I have had the joy of seeing many sick bodies healed as we have prayed believing . . . and the sick beginning a new obedience unto God. Blessed are they to whom the Lord gives faith for miracles and for divine healing; the first instantaneous, the latter gradual.

However, much reproach has been brought upon these truths because, after having been healed, the individual has failed to realize that God has given *laws* that must be observed in order to constantly maintain radiant health and a strong body. We will deal with this in the following chapter.

Most of us have heard of someone who was prayed for and from every evidence was divinely, and in some cases, miraculously healed; then, sometime later the sickness returned and a trip to the hospital and an operation were necessary. Statistics make it impossible to dismiss the first healing as "mental." What is the answer? "There is a law." Consider this with me in the next chapter.

4

There Is a Law

"There ought to be a law," we often hear the phrase. Well, there *is* a law in every realm and at every level of life. Let's take a quick glance at some of them.

For Every Effect a Cause

"For every effect there is a cause," is one of the first factual statements (learned in school) which has stuck with me through the years. Nothing just happens. As the Scriptures state, "The curse causeless shall not come" (Proverbs 26:2). As sure as life and death is the law of cause and effect. That you can repeat a certain experiment the same way and always get the same result is proof of the law of cause and effect. This law is in operation in every sphere of life.

Various Universal Laws

The entire universe is governed by law. All of life operates according to law. When we observe these laws, we get definite beneficial results. When we disregard them, we get certain evil consequences. To observe them means blessing, happiness, health and long life. To disregard them means misery, sorrow, sickness and death. And let us keep in mind that laws are no respecters of persons; rejecting them does not cancel the penalty of violation even though the rejecter may appear to be very spiritual and knowledgeable.

Why was the law given? "That ye may live, and that it may be well with you, and that ye may prolong your days" (Deuteronomy 5:33; given in greater detail in Deuteronomy 28).

The laws of God were never given to bestow upon man eternal life, but rather to preserve and bless his earthly life. His salvation and forgiveness of sins came through grace. (Leviticus 17:11; See also Galatians 3:21.)

These laws, whether written or unwritten, are still in force. The law of cause and effect is operative and inviolable in every realm. For example:

(1)   In *physics,* though you had kept all other laws but disregarded *the law of gravity* and jumped off a twenty story building to the concrete below, you would suddenly reap the consequences of such a foolish action and die. Being devout and godly would not exempt you from the physical consequence. "Survivors" would soon be convinced that this law is still in force in the physical realm. Keep this in mind as we later consider God's dietary law.

(2)   In the realm of *agriculture,* the farmer knows from experience that laws govern his crops. He who sows wheat reaps the same, and so with all other grains, vegetables, fruits, nuts, etc. Crying, screaming and praying for a field that has been sown with oats to come up into stalks of corn will only reveal the folly of the fool. There is a law . . . God's law . . . and it cannot be broken. We, in disobedience, merely break ourselves over it.

(3)   In *electronics,* engineers and electricians must first not only learn the laws of their skill, but must be taught to observe them to the letter. We have known of men working on high voltage power lines who, in ignorance or

carelessness, disregarded a law of electricity. They loved life, their families and the enjoyments of this earth as much as anyone could, but they disregarded a law and were instantly killed. To think that we can change these laws by our own reasoning and disregard them even for an instant, only meets with disaster.

(4) Scientists can tell how profound are the laws of *chemistry:* In a town in Iowa a number of years ago lived a family with twin daughters. During a severe illness they contacted the family doctor who gave a prescription that was most certain to work their recovery. During the night, the mother got up and, in the semi-darkness, in order not to awaken the rest of the family, administered the medicine to the girls. The next morning, not hearing any sounds from the girls, she believed the medicine had worked a cure, but when she went into their room she found them both lifeless in bed. She screamed and went into hysterics, crying, "The doctor murdered my babies." When the doctor arrived, he discovered the medicine bottle had never been uncorked. The mother, in the semi-darkness, had taken the wrong bottle and had given her daughters poison. A law of chemistry had been broken, which resulted in the death of her girls, whom she loved so much.

A few days after the girls' funeral, there was a third mound beside theirs, that of the mother. What caused the tragedy? A broken law.

(5) God has laid down laws in *biology* that cannot be broken, fortunately. This is the reason we never see an animal that is half dog and half cat. We may twist this law temporarily to the extent of mixing a donkey with a horse to produce a mule, but the mule will not breed. There is a law.

Illustrations could be multiplied in the various fields of science, such as *physiology, hygiene, botany, chemistry, zoology, astronomy.* God's laws are in operation in all, including our orbiting rockets and satellites into space. All must operate according to the fixed laws of the Almighty, our Redeemer, "In whom are hid all the treasures of wisdom and knowledge" (Colossians 2:3). According to the prophetic Scriptures, God will allow a vast increase in learning which shall be among the signs prior to, and heralding, the coming of the Redeemer and Messiah. This has certainly been greatly fulfilled as recorded by the prophet Daniel, "knowledge shall be increased" (Daniel 12:4).

Then there is the realm of *civil laws* of which the Apostle Peter writes, "Submit yourselves to every ordinance of man for the Lord's sake" (I Peter 2:13).

And as the Apostle Paul declares in Romans 13, "Let every soul be subject unto the higher powers . . . the powers that be [governments], are ordained of God." (Read Romans 13:1–7).

Jesus declared, "Render unto Caesar the things that are Caesar's . . ." (Matthew 22:21).

How many thousands of people meet untimely deaths because they disregard traffic laws? In almost every traffic fatality on record some traffic law has been violated.

Think now of the *moral law* of God as summed up in the Ten Commandments (Exodus 20:1–17). Think of the heartache, tears and tragedies that have come to thousands who have deliberately or ignorantly disregarded these laws which God laid down for our happiness, preservation and blessing. These laws also cannot be broken: men, in violating them, merely break themselves over them.

Prisons, hospitals, mental institutions and the slums of our large cities bear stark witness to the human wreckage of society because the laws of God were disregarded. Not all of these are responsible for their sad fate, but somewhere down the line, perhaps as far back as the third or fourth generation, a law of God was thought non-essential and was transgressed—and tragedy finally resulted.

Warning to Parents

Teach your children the law of God or the police, judges and prison officials will have to do it.

"Thou shalt teach them diligently unto thy children, and shalt talk of them when thou sittest in thine house, and when thou walkest by the way, and when thou liest down, and when thou risest up" (Deuteronomy 6:7).

Impress it deeply on the minds and hearts of your sons and daughters that the laws of God cannot be broken, that in transgressing, they merely break themselves over them. Jesus also said, "The Scripture cannot be broken" (John 10:35). Warn your children to fear breaking any of the law of God as they would fear a den of hissing, poisonous rattlesnakes. Sin (transgression of the law) will reek more havoc and heartaches than any physical affliction man can know.

Then there is the *dietary law* of God, which has been ridiculed by those who thought they were wise. The world is full of those who have fallen prey to all manner of infirmity, sickness and disease—crippling and fatal—who either in ignorance or with supposed superior knowledge have disregarded the unchangeable laws of the Almighty.

5

Biblical Laws

Man's Instruction Book

While president of a home mission board in California in 1947, I served also as Director of Youth for Christ in the San Joaquin Valley area. During this time I purchased a combination disc recorder and P.A. system for use in our youth rallies.

After taking it home, I thought I should acquaint myself with its operation so I would be in the "know" when we used it. What a nerve wracking time I had. I tried every conceivable thing I knew to get a good reproduction, but no one anywhere or anytime ever made more miserable recordings. I ruined one new disc after another, starting with the inexpensive cardboard miniatures to the large professional type at $1.00 a throw. I was ready to tear my hair, take the recorder back and tell them what a miserable piece of equipment Wilcox-Gay engineers manufactured.

As a last resort I thought, "Before I do, I should get out the instruction book and see if it could help me!" Well, it did. I learned that I had the cutting needle adjustment set far too deep . . . making deep gouges in the record. I also had the tone control on bass when recordings should be made flat on treble. I had not taken the recording level electric eye into account and got distortion from having the volume too high, etc., etc. But when I followed directions I got perfect recordings.

Well, there is an instruction manual that goes with the man. Reader, do not be surprised as you talk to folk about our Maker's Instruction Book regarding building our bodies if you get an adverse attitude of "I know how to run this body . . . It doesn't matter what you eat. Those Biblical instructions are for other people (such as the Jews), not me." Be patient; sow the seed. At some later date they may need and receive the very information you gave them. Many *will* accept the instruction and be saved from much of the misery and anguish that so many are suffering. I also at first rejected instruction. Now, I thank God every day I live that I have this knowledge which has blessed me with health and strength for over 40 years.

The Three Classes of Biblical Laws

Before exploring the dietary law, it is essential that we have a basic understanding of the three types of laws given by the Almighty. This is foundational. Don't just skim through it.

The Eternal God declares:

"Let us hear the conclusion of the whole matter: Fear God, and keep his commandments: for this is the whole duty of man" (Ecclesiastes 12:13).

"To the law and to the testimony; if they speak not according to this word, it is because there is no light in them" (Isaiah 8:20).

"He that turneth away his ear from hearing the law, even his prayer shall be abomination" (Proverbs 28:9).

The laws of God recorded in the Hebrew Scriptures can generally be classified into three categories:

1. *The moral law*, with its many ramifications, summed up in the Ten Commandments (Exodus 20:1–17; Deuteronomy 5:7–21).

2. *The dietary law* (Leviticus 11 and Deuteronomy 14:3–21).

3. *The ceremonial law* (Exodus 25 through 40 and the book of Leviticus).

All of these laws were given by the Creator to Moses for His people Israel, as a guide to the nations. Stern penalties for violators were attached to give laws 'staying power' to avoid anarchy and for sure protection of individual rights.

1. The Almighty held up a perfect standard of righteousness in *the moral law:* "An eye for an eye, a tooth for a tooth, and life for life" (Exodus 21:24 and Leviticus 24:20).

2. Diseases of the heathen nations would be visited upon those who disregarded *the dietary law:* "Whereof thou canst not be healed" (Deuteronomy 28:27,35).

3. *The ceremonial law* that set forth the Messiah in its various embodiments which was to be kept to the letter "was the figure for the time then present" (Hebrews 9:1–9).

There is some confusion and question as to what a Christian's attitude should be toward the law. Some raise the cry of "legalism" to those who have obedient respect for God's law. Others, without doubt, are enslaved to the law, believing its perfect obedience is essential to eternal salvation (Romans 3:19–28; 4:5; Galatians 2:16, etc.). Some believe we should observe parts of it as a moral code, such as the Ten Commandments. Others believe the law of tithing is still in force, and fragments of commandments though only briefly referred to in passing in connection with other subjects in the New Testament. Some claim if it is not mentioned in the New Testament, it should be rejected: Because "Thou shalt not take the name of the Lord thy God in vain" is not in the New Testament, is it right then to curse God? What is the true Scriptural position?

Consider: God *being perfect and righteous* could only make a perfect, righteous law, and *being perfectly just* He must demand the total penalty for the breaking of such a law. *Man* being *imperfect* and *unrighteous* cannot keep such a righteous law perfectly and therefore falls under the *total penalty* that the *justice* of God demands.

Herein lies the gospel (good news): Christ kept all of *the moral law* and *the dietary law* perfectly, and He *was* the embodiment and fulfillment of *the ceremonial law,* and so, observed the whole law, beginning with His circumcision on the eighth day to the end of His life when He could stand before the throngs of people and query, "Which of you convinceth me of sin?"—transgressing the law?

Christ became the personification of the righteousness of the law *perfectly fulfilled.* The *law* cannot condemn Him or exact the penalty from Him. If He would have been judged according to the justice of the *law,* He would have been set free. He would never have descended into death and hell but would have been caught up immediately into the Glory. Yet He went to the cursed tree and died an ignominious, criminal death. Why? . . . To demonstrate His infinite love for us and to perform the work of redemption. God is not only *righteous* and *just* but also *merciful* and full of loving kindness and compassion.

Here at the cross, mercy and justice are met together in Christ, righteousness and peace have kissed each other. Hallelujah! The condemnation of the broken law is lifted because Christ has borne its guilt and penalty.

What a tragedy today that the nations still reject Christ, and needlessly carry this heavy burden of guilt on their own souls which robs them of the knowledge of life eternal, peace and true joy, when our Redeemer purchased all for them.

Israel should be a special object of our love and understanding, especially at this point of prophetic history as the nations (U.N.) turn against them. As Joseph revealed himself to his brethren after becoming Prime Minister of Egypt (a type of 'the world'), so Messiah-Christ will reveal Himself to His brethren

(Israel) on His return to reign as King of kings in Jerusalem. At the present, "They, not understanding God's righteousness [Christ], and going about to establish their own righteousness, have not submitted themselves unto the righteousness of God. For Christ is the end of the law for righteousness to everyone that believeth" (Romans 10:3,4). To realize "concerning the gospel they are enemies for your sakes. . . ." and that we "have now obtained mercy through their unbelief," should humble us and intensify our love and compassion for them (Romans 11:28–31).

To sum up then: Christ kept all of the *moral law,* the *dietary law* and He was the fulfillment of the *ceremonial law.* Now all of this (His) righteousness, dazzling in brilliance and glorious in its perfection is charged to our account because we receive Him, Christ, as our Messiah-Redeemer, as our substitute who paid the death penalty for our transgressions of the law.

"There is therefore now no condemnation to them which are in Christ Jesus . . . For the law of the spirit of life in Christ Jesus hath made me free from the law of sin and death—for what the law could not do through physical weakness . . . God sending His own Son in the likeness of sinful flesh, and for sin, condemned sin in the flesh that the righteousness of the law might be fulfilled in us who walk not after the flesh but after the Spirit" (Romans 8:1–4, slightly paraphrased).

As far as salvation and eternal life are concerned, the believer is not to be in bondage under the law. Christ paid the penalty of our violation (Galatians 3:10–13). Christ died our death and bore away our eternal punishment. We now are dead, legally, before God through Christ's death—reckon it so, Paul writes —but also eternally alive through His resurrection. (Romans 6:11.)

The *soul* is redeemed through Christ's sacrificial death, but Paul speaks for us all when he says that "We groan within ourselves, waiting for . . . the redemption of our *body*" (Romans 8:23). As long as we live in this body, we must realize that it is subject to all the physical laws that God laid down for its normal function and well-being. When this body shall be changed and "fashioned like unto His glorious body" (Philippians 3:21), and at His appearance when "we shall be like Him" (I John 3:2), we can then forget all these laws that God made for our welfare in this present world.

What should be the Christian's attitude now toward the law? I believe it is very plain. Because of Christ's work, we are dead . . . legally . . . reckon it so. Now yield yourself, your body, mind and soul to Christ who alone could keep the law, and let His Spirit, working in you, fulfill the righteousness of the law through you. In other words, Christ by His Spirit will be in you giving direction and strength to live a righteous life. He not only puts the desire within you to want to keep God's law, but His Spirit actually does it for you as you yield to Him.

The Law of the Spirit

"For it is God that worketh in you both to will and to do of His good pleasure" (Philippians 2:13). This is the new covenant (testament) that God promised Israel in Jeremiah 31:31–34 and as Paul relates in Hebrews 8:10, ". . . I will put my laws in their minds, and write them in their hearts. . . ."

There is another Bible law called, "The law of the Spirit of life in Christ Jesus." It is one that makes us free from the law of sin and death. No wonder this message of Christ is called, *"Good news"* (gospel). Christ now *is* our *salvation,* our *righteousness* and our *eternal life* (I John 5:9–13). And, "He that hath the Son, hath life." Hallelujah! Reader, if you do not have the assurance of this life eternal, will you this very moment believe and act upon the promise God has given? "That if thou shalt confess with thy mouth the Lord Jesus [Jesus as Lord], and shalt believe in thine heart that God hath raised Him from the dead, thou shalt be saved" ['delivered'—from every negative force]—Romans 10:9. (An unexplainable mystery but gloriously 'functional.')

There are some who have seemingly believed on Christ but have taken a careless attitude toward His holy law; i.e., saying, by example and precept, that we need not be too careful in obeying and walking in it. Some, in order to cover their inconsistent lives, lightly lip, "I am not under law, but under grace." These shall find to their sorrow and shame that the laws of God are still in force regarding our earthly walk and conduct. The Lord *does* take us to heaven on the merits of His own righteousness apart from the law; but now the love of Messiah within should constrain us to walk in His law, for it is written in our minds and on our hearts.

We need a right and solemn glimpse of the cross to get God's true concept of righteousness and of the 'broken' law. It was man's transgression of the law that brought Christ to earth; for this reason He bore the shame, transgression and eternal death penalty of us all (I John 2:2). And for this cause our Lord "made himself of no reputation, took upon him the form of a servant, and was made in the likeness of men: And being found in fashion as a man, he humbled himself, and became obedient unto death, even the death of the cross" (Philippians 2:7,8). No true Christian will take the attitude—"Because Christ died, paid the penalty of the broken moral law, now I can disregard and flout it." Such a concept is moral suicide.

What should we as Christians conclude our Scriptural position to be regarding the law? Should not Christ be our standard and example in all matters of faith, conduct and practice (Romans 6:11—8:4)? Christ honored and kept all of God's wonderful law or He could not have been our sin-bearer. Let us accept this free and glorious gift of salvation, and then seek in all our ways to follow His example by walking in God's protective and happiness-producing law. Never did Christ do less than the law, but many times went beyond it (Matthew 5). Let us be followers of Him in this also, by God's attendant mercies, but let us never be found in the ranks of the lawless and disobedient. "And hereby we do know that we know him, if we keep his commandments. He that saith, I know him, and keepeth not his commandments, is a liar, and the truth is not in him . . . He that saith he abideth in him ought himself also so to walk, even as he walked" (I John 2:3,4,6). It was essential that He walk in all the law of God perfectly or He could not have been the sinless sacrifice.

Let us now come to grips with the controversy regarding the dietary law. Some contend this was given only to Israel. But the moral law (Ten Commandments) was also given to Israel at the same time and on the same level. On what grounds can we treat one differently than the other? As the *moral law* was given for the *moral welfare* of the people, so the *dietary law* was given for their *physical well-being.* Only the ceremonial law, given in shadows, symbols and figures, such as the candles, showbread, lamb, etc., was a type of the Messiah, and eternal salvation. On what grounds, then, dare we reject the dietary law? There is none.

All of God's law is still in force regarding this earthly life. As Jesus said, it cannot be broken (John 10:35). I repeat; we merely break ourselves over it. Consider with me God's dietary law in this next chapter.

6

God's Dietary Law

Warning note: Those with weak stomachs should not read this chapter immediately before or after meals!!

Let's now consider this dietary law prescribed to us by the Great Physician, the Almighty, as found in Leviticus chapter 11, and Deuteronomy 14. Read it carefully. Here are some concerted excerpts.

Divine Instructions

"These are the beasts which ye shall eat among all the beasts that are on the earth" (verse 2).

"Whatsoever parteth the hoof, and is clovenfooted, and cheweth the cud, among the beasts, that shall ye eat" (verse 3).

"Nevertheless these shall ye not eat of them that chew the cud, or of them that divide the hoof; as the camel, because he cheweth the cud, but divideth not the hoof; he is unclean unto you" (verse 4).

Then follows one of America's favorite delicacies: "And the swine [pig], though he divide the hoof, and be clovenfooted, yet he cheweth not the cud; he is unclean to you" (verse 7).

"Of their flesh shall ye not eat, and their carcass shall ye not touch; they are unclean to you" (verse 8).

"These shall ye eat of all that are in the waters: whatsoever hath fins and scales in the waters, in the seas, and in the rivers, them shall ye eat" (verse 9).

"And all that have not fins and scales in the seas, and in the rivers, of all that move in the waters, and of any living thing which is in the waters, they shall be an abomination unto you" (verse 10).

"They shall be even an abomination unto you; ye shall not eat of their flesh, but ye shall have their carcasses in abomination" (verse 11).

"Whatsoever hath no fins nor scales in the waters, that shall be an abomination unto you" (verse 12).

Then the various clean and unclean fowl are mentioned.

Clean and Unclean Meat Manufacture

The clean animals that chew the cud and have divided hoof such as the ox, sheep, goat, deer, cow, steer, buffalo, etc., because of the sacculated condition of the alimentary canal and the secondary cud receptacle, have practically three stomachs as refining agencies and cleansing laboratories for purifying their food. This cleanses their systems of all poisonous and deleterious matter. It takes their clean vegetable food over *twenty-four hours* to be turned into flesh, which flesh even the pre-Mosaic law said was clean. This was not mere "ceremonial" cleansing, but it was made hygienically and physiologically clean and wholesome.

In comparison, we find that the swine's (hog's) anatomy, as a supplement to his bad appetite (eating any putrid thing he finds), has but one poorly constructed stomach arrangement, and very limited excretory organs generally. Consequently, in about *four hours* after the pig has eaten his polluted swill and other putrid, offensive matter, man may eat the same second-handed off the ribs of the pig.

Some ask, "Why did the Lord make the unclean animals?" They were created as scavengers; as a rule they are meat-eating animals that clean up anything that is left dead in the fields, etc. If a dog (or any animal whatsoever) should die in the field and lie in the sun and bloat, until it is broken open and the maggots and putrefaction have set in, then the swine or other scavengers will come and eat up all this filth and putrid matter, thereby keeping disease germs from spreading over the earth and killing off mankind. But scavengers were never created for human consumption.

The God-given Mosaic law condemns this meat, manufactured out of the filthiest and most abominable matter, as *unclean*. In its very nature it is poisonous, diseased and deadly. The flesh of the swine is said by many authorities to be the prime cause of much of our American ill health, causing blood diseases, weakness of the stomach, liver troubles, eczema, consumption, tumors, cancer, etc.

It is also essential for our own welfare to observe the dietary law regarding the clean fish identified by fins and scales. Among these we have a large variety of such fish as the bass, pike, sunfish, perch, salmon, tuna, etc. The scaleless fish and all shell fish including the oyster, clam, lobster, shrimp, etc., modern science discovers to be but lumps of devitalized and disease-producing filth, because of inadequate excretion. These are the scavengers, "the garbage containers," of the waters and the seas.

The unclean fowl which are prohibited are named in the dietary law, as given in Leviticus chapter II. Some fowl such as geese, ducks, chickens and turkeys are clean by virtue of the gizzard that separates and cleanses all matter before it becomes flesh.

Why are some so naive as to pay exorbitant fees for dietetic advice, given by imperfect dietitians who are limited in knowledge, while rejecting a perfect nutritional program given so freely by an all-wise and all-knowing, infallible Creator who designed and made our bodies? We are aware that special pre-scribed diets by expert physicians are many times helpful and necessary, but there is evidence that even these could eventually be eliminated if the Scriptural dietary law were adhered to strictly. Let us follow the counsel of the Chief Nutritionist, our Lord Himself.

Disguised Garbage

Since with so many, especially for breakfast, hog is the num-ber one choice meat dish of all the unclean beasts (don't know why they slight the rats, skunks, dogs, and cats, but swine do get bigger and have large litters and so make more filthy lucre), let us consider the diet of this 'tasty' palate tickler.

Mr. John Johnson of Williams, Iowa, a farmer, speaks on this subject. He states that the swine in Iowa are principally fed on corn, but "will eat anything we give them. If anything dies, we throw it to the hogs. I have actually seen hogs chewing at the cancer of other hogs and these hogs are shipped to market. Many times cattle are infected from the incurable diseases of the hog called the 'mad itch.' It is transmitted by the hog's saliva left on the corn which cattle eat. The itching in the cattle becomes so intense they will run from stump to stump until they rub their skin from their mouths and soon die. When the saliva from the hog's mouth will poison cattle in this way, how can hogs be fit for man to eat?"

While conducting a revival campaign in Litchfield, Min-nesota, the pastor of the church told me of one of his members who raised hogs. At regular periods this farmer would go to the poultry hatchery and load his trailer full of the old rotten eggs that hadn't hatched, many with dead chicks (in various stages) in them. This, of course, would make a gooey, oozing, bloody, stinking mess.

Sometimes this farmer would stop by the parsonage and the pastor stated the smell was so horrible and "stunk up the neighborhood" so badly, that it was a source of real embarrassment to the pastor. The farmer would feed this decayed, rotten, stinking substance to his hogs. And remember, what a hog eats is on his bones in four hours and ready for consumption by ... you? This family's primary meat dish was this swine. It was no wonder to me when I learned of the constant and various illnesses in that household.

If swine are raised in a feed lot with other animals such as the horse, the cow, etc., they will eat and drink the very refuse of these animals. This is a common occurrence on farms where the animals are not separated.

While on vacation as a boy at Cotesfield, Nebraska, I remember visiting a family who were farmers. I noticed the wife of my host kept a slop bucket where she dumped all sorts of refuse, sour matter, rotten tomatoes, garbage, dirty dish water and anything they couldn't eat. She would then take this down to the pig pen and "slop the hogs." How they loved it. In a few days they slaughtered the hogs and started putting all these second-hand "delicate cuts" on the table in its various forms.

I could just never figure out what made slop good for human consumption because a hog ate it. Does feeding rotten, filthy garbage (maggots and all) to a hog sanctify and cleanse it as some would have us believe? Did anything biologically happen to the swine when Christ died? Or did the digestive tract of man have some kind of miracle transformation? No, the Bible, science, and experience have all proven the contrary.

What's in Crops Out

The hog is still unclean. Swine actually have "running sores" under their hoofs. To prove it to yourself, visit a farm sometime where they are raised. Lift the front hoof of the hog and with just a little pressure you will find greenish matter oozing out from between his "toes." This is one small outlet for the various heinous poisons that he takes into his body. Sometimes this artery becomes stopped up and the poison backs up into his system and greenish growths are formed in various parts of his body.

During a campaign in south Minnesota, the leader of the young people's society told me that he had worked only a few days at a certain meat packing plant that summer and he had seen hogs come down the line with big greenish growths on them. He said, "We were instructed to just trim them off and when the meat inspector came he put his stamp of approval upon them." Such statements have been made also by others who have worked in meat packing plants.

"Death in the Pot"

While in this same area in Minnesota, I had the opportunity of visiting a mink farm which was owned by one of the members of my host church. This mink raiser, who knew his business said, "If we fed pork or any part of the swine to our mink, they would die. We feed them horse meat and they thrive on it, but without exception after eating pork products they sicken and die." On this certain mink farm they bought old broken down horses and used an average of three a day.

Moral: If you have a choice, better eat horse meat instead of swine, if you prefer health and life to sickness and death. Though a horse is in the unclean category, it is a vegetarian and doesn't eat all the vile, gory refuse that a hog revels in. Stop and consider.

The following story is on court record. The Silver Moon Mink Farm of New Holstein, Wisconsin, owned by the Langenfeldts, ordered a supply of beef livers for their mink from a meat packing plant. Instead, the packers shipped them pork livers unbeknown to the Langenfeldts, who fed them to the mink. What was the result? *All the mink died.* Yes, there was a lawsuit and the meat packers had to pay. Let the mink teach us a lesson. Shouldn't we be more discriminating about our diet than a glorified weasel?

This story from Florida was told me by a native son of that sunshine state. "Whenever we have a snake infested area in Florida, we just turn the hogs loose on them," he related. "The only animal that a snake is afraid of is the hog. The swine are so full of poison, the snakes cannot kill them but the hogs kill and eat the snakes." Brother, if you still want your ham, help yourself. 'Fools rush in where serpents fear to tread.'

"Can't we eat pork and still go to heaven?" people have asked me.

"Sure," I answer, "you might even go a little quicker."

As we were taking a guided tour through a meat packing house in Minnesota, a slaughterer told me they use every part of the hog; nothing is wasted . . . pork chops, ham, bacon, the intestines for sausages and wieners, head cheese of the head, pickle the feet, brains, liver, the hide for bacon rind and salt pork, etc. (Wieners and lunch meats, unless specified as beef, are mostly made of the worst trimmings of pork and other meats.) "There is only one thing that we do not utilize in the hog," he said, "and that is the 'grunt.' " I couldn't help saying, "That isn't lost either, brother, the swine-eater will get plenty of 'grunts' and groans before the final 'countdown.' "

The following word comes from the Almighty's capital city of Jerusalem, Israel:

Israel's parliament approved by a vote of 42 to 15 a ban on pig-raising in Israel. It prohibited the "raising, keeping or slaughtering" of swine except in Nazareth and six other places which have a large Christian population (that demand the unclean diet!)—a sad commentary on heathen customs of those supposedly 'enlightened.' Both Jewish and Moslem religious law forbids eating of hogs.

The new law allowed swine farmers a year to dispose of their present holdings of pigs. After that date, anyone caught raising the animals, except for scientific purposes or display in zoos, faced a fine of 1,000 Israel pounds. Renting of premises for a pig sty carried a fine of 500 pounds. Former Prime Minister, Mr. David Ben-Gurion of Israel, stated at the Jubilee Celebration of Israel's Medical Association that, "Israel has the lowest death rate in the world" [i.e., the highest life expectancy]. Could this merely be chance, or the fulfillment of God's promises? "If thou wilt diligently hearken to the voice of the Lord thy God, and wilt do that which is right in his sight, and wilt give ear to his commandments, and keep all his statutes, I will put none of these diseases upon thee, which I have brought upon the Egyptians: for I am the Lord that healeth thee" (Exodus 15:26). Without question it is because the people of Israel, as a whole, observe the dietary law of God, which insures them against untold physical affliction, disease and premature death.

Operation Goldswine

For several summers it was our privilege to have the Jim Van Koevering family as guests in our home. They were for years known as the "Swiss Bell Ringers" of St. Petersburg, Florida, and as a family played a host of well known and many unique musical instruments.

Mr. James Van Koevering, before his conversion, was in the

professional show business. He counted such personalities as
Mr. Edgar Bergen among his close friends. To a degree, his
early life paralleled that of Mel Trotter, under whose ministry
he surrendered his life to God for full time Christian service,
and they became lifelong friends. (Mel Trotter's marvelous and
transforming conversion to Christ—from chief drunkard—was
instrumental in his becoming the "Father" of city rescue mis-
sions across America.)

Mrs. Van Koevering told us the following true story of a
relative who lived in the state of Michigan. Mr. H. owned a
farm on which there were some deep ravines which he wished
to fill. Then he came on a very brilliant idea. He invested in a
herd of hogs and a few trucks and contracted for a garbage
route in the nearby town. The garbage dumped in the ravines
supplied more than ample feed for the swine.

This was a wonderful arrangement and soon became a real
"goldswine." Why hadn't someone thought of it before? They
had: It is a common practice wherever pagan eating habits exist.
He really began to prosper—financially. Almost immediately
there was a big income with minimum expense. He bought
more trucks, increased his garbage route, and bought more
trucks and more hogs and the hogs bore more pigs. They had
the world by the (pig) tail.

Soon, however, neighbors began to complain. The hog farm
was not only an "eye sore" but a "nose sore" as well. The
obnoxious stench was more than Farmer Patience could endure. The result? Mr. H. bought his neighbor's farm. The vile
odor got worse and spread to other farms. He bought their
farms, too. Finally irritated citizens said the place was a public
nuisance because of having to endure the loathsome stench
while driving by the hog haven. The outcome? He bought the
road leading by his farms. Nothing seemed to hinder his onward march of prosperity until. . . .

Mr. H. began having trouble keeping drivers for his trucks. They would work for awhile and get sick and have to quit. This problem continued and got worse, which at times all but halted the "goldswine" operation. (Why did the drivers get sick? They also ate the hogs fattened on this garbage.)

Mr. H. had secured two beautiful, husky, German shepherd watch dogs in the beginning of this project to guard against prowlers and thieves. At the start, they were unusually alert and active. They not only got scraps but special portions of the swill-fed swine were prepared for them. In a relatively short time these fine dogs began to lose weight, became listless and just wanted to lie around and do nothing but sleep. It was not long until they finally sickened and died. This was not the worst.

Mr. H. and his family became ill more and more frequently. Doctor and hospital bills mounted. They began to suffer from various and rare ailments. Children that were born to them were found to have these diseases from birth. They were spending more and more for medical and hospital treatment in their search for relief and health. At last, it was necessary for them to sell their farm and move to Arizona where doctors recommended that they seek help and benefit from the more direct healing rays of the sun. We sincerely hope their ailments have been arrested or even completely cured.

Some contend that since many cities now require that garbage fed to 'stockyard-hogs' must be cooked, it minimizes the danger of trichinosis——it is supposed to kill the poisonous little trichinae worms. We reiterate, who wants to eat dead, poisonous worms? Others say that corn-fed hogs must be perfectly safe! But what farmer would hire someone to 'police' his hogs 24 hours each day to see that they did not eat dead rats or snakes or any other maggot-infested deleterious matter found on the place? Who could offer a certified guarantee? But above all we should follow the Eternal's dietary law because He decreed it, i.e., in order to please Him and to be obedient to His Word. "I am the Lord, I change not." This is the prime reason observant Jews keep the dietary law—should we do less? Why should we forever be on the stretch to see how many command-ments we can 'break' without getting hurt? Why shouldn't we 'hug the mountain' instead of seeing how close we can get to the edge of the precipice before falling off?

Clean Inside and Out

We have heard some say, "I've eaten pork (swine) all my life and it hasn't hurt me." But do they know how much sharper and in more vibrant health they might have been had they honored God's Word? I heard of a baby that fell from a fast moving train and, to the amazement of all, they found the infant without a scratch. Is the moral of this story to start throwing babies out of moving trains? We have heard of thieves who operated for years without being caught. Does this prove steal-ing is right? May the Spirit of God open our hearts to receive and obey His truth for our blessing and God's glory.

A personal friend of mine who was proprietor-owner of a supermarket and also an expert butcher, gave me a very perti-nent fact about meat. He stated, "When pork begins to get bad, it spoils from the inside out, where it is noticed last. On the other hand," he said, "when beef breaks down, it starts on the outside. This can be trimmed off and the inside is just as good as ever." This is another corroboration of the wisdom of the dietary law.

Should we not conclude that the Chief Nutritionist and *Great Physician* (headquarters, Heaven) knew what He was doing when He separated the clean animals from the unclean for our physical health and well-being? Let us abide by His prognosis and prescribed health plan.

When our Lord reminds us that "Ye are the temple of the living God," He is talking about our bodies; and He continues, "I will dwell in them and walk in them [their bodies], and I will be their God, and they shall be my people. Wherefore, come out from among them, and be ye separate, saith the Lord, and touch not the unclean thing. . . ." Here God declares that He wants to dwell and walk in clean bodies . . . is yours? We prefer to spiritualize these passages, but God is talking about *our bodies,* which the context proves, "and I will receive you, and will be a Father unto you, and ye shall be my sons and daughters, saith the Lord Almighty." Unfortunately the chapter divides there, for the next verse is related, "Having therefore these promises, dearly beloved, let us cleanse ourselves from all filthiness of the flesh and spirit, perfecting holiness in the fear of God" (II Corinthians 6:16–7:1). Let us allow God to say what He means.

Many who profess to live holy lives would never defile God's temple with cigarettes or hard liquors, but will take second-hand, disease-laden, maggot-infested garbage into these temples of God and still boldly contend they are keeping the temple clean. I reiterate, what thinking person can believe that all this vile refuse is sanctified and made clean because a hog has eaten it?

The Apostle Paul inspired by God's Spirit writes, "Be not conformed [to the heathen . . . but rather to] the perfect will of God." Which shall we choose—good or evil, clean or unclean, holy or unholy? Your future welfare hangs in the balance.

I am keenly aware of the weight of prejudice produced through centuries of common acceptance of pagan eating habits. The adoption of heathen (those who know not God) customs, on the part of Christians, is not isolated to diet, but is evident in fashions, desecration of the Lord's Day and in other areas.

We live in a day of "carbon copies," of conformity. "What monkey sees, monkey does." There are few "Abrahams" and many "Lots," few great Christians with strong convictions. "Follow the crowd," is the order of the day, but "if the blind lead the blind, both shall fall into the ditch" (Matthew 15:14) and the "ditches" are full.

7

Trichinosis, the Subtle Killer

A Scientist Speaks

Trichinosis is the name of the disease that originates with the trichina worm. (The scientific term is *trichinella spiralis.*) The trichina is one of eighteen or nineteen worms found in swine (hogs), not to mention lice or other diseases such as rickets, the thumps, mange, etc. The trichina worm is deadly. Let's listen to a scientific expert in this field:

In the 1950 March issue of *Reader's Digest,* Laird S. Goldsborough writes, "In the pork which we Americans eat, there too often lurk myriads [countless numbers] of baffling and sinister parasites. They are minute spiral worms which scientists call *Trichinella spiralis.*" He continues, "a single serving of infected pork—even a single mouthful—can kill or cripple or condemn the victim to a lifetime of aches and pains." For this unique disease, trichinosis, there is no sure cure—no drug to stop them (not even in 1976).

Dr. Goldsborough's article goes on to say, "In the flesh of a pig, the trichinae are often so minute and so nearly transparent that, to find them, even with a microscope, is a task for expert scientific inspectors. . . . Remember this: When you see stamped on a pork product the words, 'U.S. Government Inspected and Passed,' those words do not mean that any official inspection whatever has been made as to whether this pork is trichinous or not. It has merely passed the routine inspection given meat in general." (Regulations as of 1976.)

Notables Warn

London's eminent Sir James Paget, who discovered this parasite in 1835, wrote: "Fancy the body of a single individual supporting more separately existing creatures than the whole population of the world!" Seems impossible? This word comes from a specialist.

Dr. Maurice C. Hall, as Chief of the Division of Zoology of the U.S. Public Health Service, commented, "It appears to be a legitimate demand that, when a man exchanges dollars for pork, he should not do it on the basis that he may be purchasing his death warrant," speaking in regard to the infected meat of the swine.

Senator Thomas C. Desmond, who served as chairman of the New York Trichinosis Commission stated, "Physicians have confused trichinosis with some *fifty ailments,* ranging from typhoid fever to acute alcoholism." Continuing he states, "That pain in your arm or leg may be arthritis or rheumatism, but it may be trichinosis; that pain in your back may mean a gall-bladder involvement, but it may mean trichinosis."

It has been reported from a lab of one of our northern universities that trichinae-laden swine flesh was heated to an unbelievably high temperature and then put under a microscope. To the amazement of the technicians some worms were still alive and moving about. The supposition that all of these worms can be killed in cooking is not to be relied upon. Why take a chance with such a crippler and killer?

In another scientific laboratory, examinations were made of the joints of arthritic swine. The exact formation and build-up of arthritic cells were found in the swine as is common in the arthritis in humans. Did the pigs get it from people or people from pigs?

Other Dangers

The trichina is just one worm found in the swine. There is a large round worm, the gullet worm, three kinds of stomach worms, a tiny hair worm, a hookworm and the thorn-headed worm, in the small intestine. There are several species of nodular worms and one species of whip worm in the large intestine, and the kidney worm. The large round worm can be as long as eighteen inches. (Dr. Hess and Clark in "The Barnyard Doctor," Ashland, Ohio).

Could it be, since physicians have confused their diagnosis of trichinosis with fifty different ailments, that this worm could be the cause of one of the great killers in America today—cancer? My personal belief is that it is one of the great causes of this dreaded disease which I will touch on in the next chapter.

As I picked up the *Kansas City Times* one morning, I noticed a headline on the front page which read, "Big Swine Kill," and the next line, "To stamp out disease." The article went on to state that 4,900 hogs had to be destroyed because they were infected with *vesicular exanthema,* a disease in hogs similar to the hoof and mouth disease which is found occasionally in cattle.

The female trichina, greatly enlarged, showing the evolution of her eggs into the emerging young. The smaller worm is the male which dies after the female is fertilized.

The hogs were owned by the B Construction Company, holder of the city garbage collection contract. This means they bought all the garbage collected in Kansas City and used it to fatten the hogs that they had bought from farmers throughout the Midwest. Only a fraction of the imagination is required to realize that decomposed garbage 'covers a multitude of offensive corruption.' When a veterinarian was called, he diagnosed the virus infection immediately and quarantined all the other animals. The agriculture department officials asserted the disease was traceable to garbage-fed hogs.

Why do people insist on eating filthy garbage second-hand in animals that are subject to such perilous diseases? Even if these scavengers were not on the Creator's blacklist, the knowledge scientists have given us, knowing the swine to be a mobile garbage-disposal unit, should be enough to warn us of the danger of its use as a food.

(A household appliance company sent out fancy pamphlet questionnaires to housewives asking the question, "What make of garbage disposal unit do you use?" One woman answered, "Four hogs.")

In the same paper and under the same date I noticed another headline entitled, "Faces thirty years in jail." This article went on to state that an "Illinois ex-official pleads guilty in a horse meat scandal." He confessed to six indictments growing out of horse meat violations. Immediately he became liable to fines totaling $12,000 and jail or prison sentences aggregating thirty years.

Compare these two articles:

Both, according to the Scriptures, were peddling unclean meat. The first would have been guilty (had a veterinarian not stopped the selling) of starting an epidemic of a dreadful disease. He was merely detained temporarily from his money-making project. The second faced a $12,000 fine and a thirty-year prison sentence though no disease was found in the horse meat.

In the first case the swine is a far filthier animal than the horse; no great study or scientific knowledge is needed to come to such a conclusion.

The herbivorous horse feeds on grass, hay, etc., and is a much cleaner animal in every way. But in our courts the filthy carnivorous swine takes precedence because we have commonly accepted the heathen dietary customs, and because it's a fast money-maker on the market.

Several years ago a government meat inspector told the owner of a meat locker plant at Granada, Minnesota, "If the dates on the packaged pork products run past a specified given date, I must condemn all the meat in the locker." Isn't this a warning and a commentary on the Scripture that God gave regarding swine? "Their carcass shall ye not touch, they are unclean to you" (Leviticus 11:8).

Why, with all of our advances in the various fields of science and social uplift, do we retain these filthy pagan foods and deleterious dining customs that foster so many deadly and crippling diseases? Why do we have such a twisted sense of values as these above articles reveal? We are supposed to be an enlightened, Bible-believing, God-fearing nation and yet we reject the truths of the Book that we claim to believe.

Counting the Cost

"The love of money is a root of all evil" (Grk., I Timothy 6:10) and it plays a far greater part in this entire question than perhaps we are ready to admit. To the farmer, hogs are known as "mortgage lifters." They thrive and fatten on all kinds of rotten refuse and can be sent to market at a good price in a relatively short time. Baby pigs come in large litters of eight, ten and twelve. It has been known for large sows to have as many as 22 baby pigs born at a time. The horse, of course, cannot be reproduced nearly as fast, so we must whet our appetite for the putrid, lucrative swine—of which the Almighty (who declares, "I change not") warns about even touching their dead carcasses (Leviticus 11:8).

We have been so thoroughly brainwashed and indoctrinated into pagan eating habits that not only have we commonly accepted a heathen diet to our hurt and destruction (Hosea 4:6), but we look with disdain and stamp the label "heretic" on anyone who is brash enough to suggest we return to the Biblical paths of clean nutrition.

Miss Joan Wells, instructor of nurses at The Wesley Medical Center, Wichita, Kansas, informed us, as we were preparing this book for the press, of a special report on trichinosis given at a Doctors and Nurses Conference on Communicable Diseases. It was very revealing:

A Dr. Manley, who is an expert on animal diseases, made the statement that autopsies showed that one out of three people are infected with trichinosis. This means there is a tremendous increase in the spread of this subtle crippler and killer.

The Lord has mercifully warned us about the diseases lurking in these unclean animals and of the perilous consequences of disobeying His commandments and statutes (Deuteronomy 28:27,35). They are God's warning signals, flashing red lights, installed in the Book of God to keep us from disaster.

Many today make sport of the God-given scientific Mosaic laws and laugh themselves right into the hospital and into a coffin. Of whom are they making light? A scientist such as Dr. Goldsborough? A minister who faithfully declares God's message? No, but it is the Almighty they are holding up to ridicule, in whose hand is their very life and breath. Fools blurt out where angels fear to whisper. These divine directives are not the arguments of a man but factual statements from the indestructible Word of the Eternal God. *Let us beware of mocking God* who gave these Words of wisdom (Proverbs 14:9).

Isaiah on Swine

It is amazing to discover to what extent the book of Isaiah with its 66 chapters parallels the 66 books of the Bible, chapter for book. This may not be carried out exactly to the letter but it can be generally in essence, beginning with Genesis 1 and Isaiah chapter 1, where God speaking forth to heaven and earth, states the result of sin upon man, then on to the new heaven and earth set forth in both Isaiah chapter 66 and Revelation 21–22.

One clear instance is Isaiah 65 and 66 which deals with the period prior to the establishing of the Messianic kingdom—the present day—and corresponds significantly with the book of the Revelation. In the light of this, consider such passages as these (addressed to this day):

"I have spread out my hands all the day unto a rebellious people, which walk in a way that was not good, after their own thoughts; A people that provoketh me to anger continually to my face; that sacrificeth in gardens, and burneth incense upon altars of brick; Which remain among the graves, and lodge in the monuments, WHICH EAT SWINE'S FLESH, and broth of ABOMINABLE THINGS is in their vessels: which say, Stand by thyself, come not near to me; for I am holier than thou [characteristic of many present day religious groups]. These are a smoke in my nose, a fire that burneth all the day. Behold, it is written before me: I will not keep silence, but will recompense, even recompense into their bosom" (Isaiah 65:2–6).

"For behold, the Lord will come with fire, and with his chariots like a whirlwind, to render his anger with fury, and his rebuke with flames of fire. For, by fire and by his sword [judgment and warfare] will the Lord plead with all flesh: and the slain of the Lord shall be many. They that sanctify themselves, and purify themselves in the garden behind one tree in the midst, EATING SWINE'S FLESH, and the abomination and the mouse, shall be consumed together, saith the Lord" (Isaiah 66:15–17).

Let us keep in mind that the Lord by His Spirit has inspired and set these passages in Holy Writ. Many today are wresting portions of Scripture from their context to their own hurt and even destruction. Let us not pass over these verses lightly because of deeply imbedded prejudices, but realize that these also shall be fulfilled. God's judgment follows disobedience.

It would be amusing if the results were not so tragic, how many will piously turn back to Old Testament portions and accept all those great comforting passages in Isaiah on peace, trust and deliverance, and yet totally disregard the above passages because of prejudice and preconceived concepts. They take great solace in "The eternal God is thy refuge and underneath are the everlasting arms" in Deuteronomy 33, but totally reject Deuteronomy 14. They accept Leviticus 17:11, but not Leviticus 11:7 and 8. How dare we do such violence to the Holy Word of God?

". . . Because it is written, Be ye holy for I am holy." (I Peter 1:16). The Apostle Peter here quotes from the 11th chapter of Leviticus, which deals entirely with the dietary law that God gave to Moses for the physical well-being of the people. Some take this verse completely out of context. Let's allow the Lord to say what He wants us to know and to do. The final authority in this book is not scientists, or even medical doctors, but the Lord God Almighty, Maker of heaven and earth, who "took on Him not the nature of angels . . . but the seed of Abraham" (Hebrews 2:16) that He might redeem us from all iniquity. He paid the full price for our transgressions of His holy law.

Because we could only be redeemed by His GRACE, let us not flout His LAW. May we never forget that it was our infractions of the law that nailed Him to the tree. He came to save man from transgression, not to give a license that he might continue IN them. We should demonstrate His grace by walking in His law because "it is written on our hearts and in our minds," (Hebrews 8:10) "and in keeping of them there is great reward" (Psalm 19:11).

Some ask, if pork products are dangerous to the health, why does the Federal Food and Drug Administration permit its sale? We may as well ask why many other products are on the market that we know are harmful.

We owe much to the Pure Food and Drug Administration as a watchdog guarding the public against many harmful products. However, it is a human organization and the best of watchdogs sometimes fail. High Christian conviction counts the body God's temple, and such things as cancer-producing cigarettes, hard liquors, and other products are harmful and yet they are accepted and sold on the public market.

In 1976 scientists issued still another warning against the dangers of pork in this wire-service story.

New York (WUP)—"Pork processed in the United States is not examined for trichinae in routine post-slaughter inspection of carcasses," scientists at the Public Health Service's Center for Disease Control have warned. They further warned that until some legislation is passed requiring proper inspection of pork for the dreaded parasite known as Trichinella Spiralis no guarantee can be given to anyone partaking of pork contracting trichinosis.

"In brief, the swine is an animal that kills. The U.S. Public Health Service in Washington has a huge file of data on the dangers of trichinosis."

8

My Brush With Cancer

Cancer, without doubt, is the most dreaded disease in America today. There are various forms of internal and external cancer. It is no respecter of organs or members of the body, but attacks the blood, bone, lungs, brain, liver and the various parts of the body. Although some progress has been made, it still baffles medical science. Serum cures have been reported in animals but results in humans are not conclusive. Research continues and we hope that a cure may soon be discovered. In this, more than in any other sphere, it is true that "an ounce of prevention is worth a ton of cure." I am fully persuaded cancer can be prevented through proper nutrition and common sense health measures.

Faced With Death

In 1936, a doctor stated that I had a carcinoma (cancer) of the stomach with all its attendant symptoms. I was wasting away and could not have lived much longer if I had continued failing as I was. Attacks of excruciating pains first began in my stomach. Many times as I drove along in my car, I would have to stop, and pull over to the side of the road and cry out to God.

Later, I felt these sharp burning pains spreading to other sections of my body: My gall bladder also became affected.

Since I could not keep even water on my stomach (sometimes up to ten days at a stretch) but would vomit it up green, I was sure I would starve to death. I dropped in weight from 155 pounds to 115. My complexion became a greenish yellow.

Arthritis plagued me so that I could not sleep at night. I could not walk on concrete without severe pain in my hips. I would walk on soft grass turf if possible when it was necessary for me to go about.

Every organ in my body seemed to quit functioning—my bowels and kidneys—and even my nails and hair quit growing. We understand that after death the hair keeps growing. Well, I was worse than dead! God only knows the misery I suffered.

My mental torture was indescribable as the result of a complete nervous breakdown. It seemed I could get no comfort from the blessings of the past. My present seemed to be a prison of misery, and there seemed to be no hope for a future as far as an earthly existence was concerned.

Unbeknown to my loved ones, I went to physician after physician, consulted specialists and was constantly in and out of medical clinics and doctors' offices. As a dying man, I grasped at every straw. I was always on the search for anyone to talk to who had experienced anything like my afflictions. I searched any book that offered the slightest hope. Expensive prescriptions, far beyond my means, helped me none. Since there seemed to be no hope, I began to plan my own funeral service.

A Promise of Hope

In final desperation, I cried to God with all my heart and soul. Every earthly helper had failed. It was then I received the promise in Psalm 107:20, "He sent His Word and healed them." I began to study the Scriptures earnestly. I found that God's original nutritional plan before the flood was for man to live on a diet of grains, vegetables, nuts, fruits, etc. One doctor informed me that red meat builds a sweet-acid that feeds cancer, so for two years I lived on a diet without red meat but supplemented my protein by eating chicken, fish, eggs, a little cheese, milk, nuts, plus fresh vegetables and fruits. One day I awoke to the realization that my physical miseries were beginning to fade away.

At this time, I was pastor at the Calvary Baptist Church of Leavenworth, Kansas. We were in the midst of a new building project that required more than the usual activities and duties of a minister. I felt the need of a greater source of protein than I was getting. As I studied the Scriptures further, I came across the dietary law, and so began to observe this plan of eating the clean meats. Before this veritable hell of sickness and misery, I was a great consumer of every form of the swine product— pork (chops and roast), ham, sausage, bacon, lunch meats and wieners (unsanctified garbage). Now I started supplementing my diet by eating the clean meats of veal, beef, lamb and even some beef bacon and beef wieners.

I continued to gain in strength and health. That has been over forty years ago. Since that time, I have never known sickness, headaches and the various multiple ailments that so many people suffer today.

Had all this merely "happened"—by chance? No, I found that God has established the universe to operate according to law in every realm, and I have found this true also in the realm of physiology—the human body. *God's plan always works.*

Learning the Hard Way

In Kansas City back in 1948, I had a similar experience to the one regarding the recorder in California that I mentioned in Chapter 5. A good friend, an agricultural specialist and wheat farmer of Johnson, Kansas, had given us a new wire recorder for our work (just before tape machines were introduced). At a special family gathering, we made a recording of various musical numbers, jargon and humor; just one of those things that can't be duplicated.

The recorder worked fine, but I discovered one thing that made me think the designing engineers had really flubbed. I found that by holding my thumb against the rewind lever, the spool would rewind so much faster. I thought out loud, "Why didn't those dumb engineers build it that way in the first place?" As I was sitting there thinking how smart I was, holding my thumb on the rewind lever, all at once there was a noise— z-z-z-i-n-g-g-g—and there was wire all over the place. Well, I did my best to salvage this treasured recording. My brother-in-law, George Philgreen, held one end of the wire in one corner; my sister, Evelyn, held a section in another corner; my nephew, Irving, still another, as I tried to retrieve the loss (of time I was saving by improving on the engineer's workmanship).

Because I had learned to operate a disc recorder, I thought I knew all about all of them. But now I conceded that it might help to take a look at the wire recorder instruction book. There I discovered that the engineers had designed brakes to work on the rewind drums to serve as a governor and keep a tension on the wire, holding it firmly in the guiding head so it would rewind evenly. My smart-alecky idea caused the equipment to run wildly out of control until the wire, jumping loosely, left the guiding head; then havoc; loss of the recording, loss of time, a tangled mess of trouble which tapped my patience.

A Manual for Man

We have to learn many things the hard way. We think we know what we want and what is right but often do not take into account the end result. We fail to follow the instruction manual and heed its warning; "O, that they were wise, that they understood this, that they would consider their latter end" (Deuteronomy 32:29).

What's the moral? Before trouble, sickness, reverses and calamity come, let's look in the instruction Book that goes with the man and discover how he is to operate in various situations. Let's consult the Chief Engineer, the Creator and Designer of the "equipment"—man's body, soul and mind.

There is not a problem or question man can propound, but what its solution and answer is found in the Book of God. The Author Himself has written in His own bona fide guarantee for the happy and smooth operation of the man, if he will follow its instruction and precepts.

"This book of the law shall not depart out of thy mouth; but thou shalt meditate therein day and night, that thou mayest observe to do according to all that is written therein; for then thou shalt make thy way prosperous, and then thou shalt have good success" (Joshua 1:8).

9

Further Search and Research

The encouragement of my gaining strength and vitality drove me into further search for the robust health that we, as God's creatures, should expect. In the years to follow, I used my body as a laboratory in which to test the Scriptural dietary laws which I found to be "functional," not merely "ceremonial." I began to slough off these various ailments and diseases in a relatively short time. However, when one has been abusing the body through wrong and "poisonous" eating for years, he cannot expect health to be restored in a matter of a few months.

The Climb Back to Health

We are told that the body renews itself (i.e., new tissues, etc.) every seven years. You can and should begin now putting sound and healthful "building blocks" into your physical house. To you who may be sick and suffering, take hope, be patient, and be glad that you have found the upward climb to health and strength. The road back to health is something like climbing a snow covered mountain. You make five or six steps of progress and then find yourself "backsliding" two or three; and then, another seven or eight steps ahead and then, slipping again two or three, which can continue for some time. Do not let this discourage you, for you are on the mend.

Keep in mind there is a real battle going on in your system, and the evil germs do not give up without a real fight. Sometimes, as in the case of the trichina worm, though nature cannot completely destroy them, she will, if given the opportunity, isolate them and wall them away from vital organs by making cysts, etc.

In my own case, the climb to health gradually became more steady, although there were times when my stomach and gall bladder would kick up, but the attacks became less frequent. Suddenly one day, after about three years, I awoke to the realization that all the miseries of aches and pains were gone. I was not bubbling over with vitality, but I knew I had fully recovered.

From that day to this (over forty years) I have never had a recurrence, but have been well and strong, never knowing what it is to have even a headache. My one exception, which can happen to the strongest, was my being poisoned by left-over spoiled chicken salad at a California drive-in, in 1947, which incapacitated me for a day. When I was relieved of that, by way of regurgitation, I was okay and on my way again.

Friends Fall Cancer Victims

After my recovery, I decided to do my own private research work. I felt I owed a debt to others who were suffering as I had, and that I must put as much information and proof in their hands as possible. I made a special point of interviewing those who had cancer.

I visited one lady about seventy years old who was filled with cancer, with running sores all over her body. She said, "Brother Elmer, why did God put this cancer on me? I have been a good, clean and moral woman. I do not understand it."

In the course of the conversation I asked, "What has been

your principal meat dish through the years?"

"Pork," she answered. "We lived on a farm where we raised hogs. That was and still is our main meat dish." (Time and again I would come to visit and she would have swine in its worst form—salt pork—frying on the stove.)

I further questioned, "What did your mother die from?"

"Cancer," she said.

And again I asked, "What was her principal meat diet?"

Again she answered, "Pork, for they raised only hogs on their farm and they lived almost solely on this meat."

This dear lady suffered excruciating distress and torment from this loathsome disease, which gradually and painfully took her life.

After leaving Leavenworth, I went to California. My first week in the sunshine state was spent in Altadena, in the home of a former pastor of Broadway Baptist (my home church) in Kansas City, Missouri. His wife had undergone an operation for cancer a number of weeks before, and now it was showing signs of further spreading. I tried to help her by telling her of my experience, and suggested that she should give up eating unclean scavenger meats, such as pork. She said, "Oh, I never eat it." (Many fail to realize it comes in many forms.) Yet the entire week that I was there, the dear lady served salt pork each morning for breakfast. She craved it so much, that after her husband had finished eating his, and had left the rind laying on his plate, she would reach over and get the rind (the hide) and chew it down. It was only a matter of a few months afterward that I received word of her death.

While conducting an evangelistic campaign one summer in Kansas City, Missouri, I talked with a woman after the service who had a huge, angry cancer on her left cheek, which was literally eating away her face. She said, "Pork is the only kind of meat I can eat. This thing hurts if I eat beef or anything else."

I am sure, reader, you can figure this out for yourself. The pork was feeding the cancer and making it feel good, even as the dope addict when he gets his dope. What a subtle, loathsome thing. Our God has warned us of this, "Whereof thou canst not be healed" (Deuteronomy 28). We have ridiculed this dietary law to our own destruction. Let us not be "fools that despise wisdom and instruction." But instead realize that "the fear of the Lord [and His Word] is the beginning of knowledge" (Proverbs 1:7).

A number of years ago a friend of mine died with cancer of the liver. Before his fatal illness he weighed about 250 pounds. He was a great lover of swine meat and pork chops in particular. He would eat as high as six or seven pork chops at a meal. The last time I saw him, he weighed about 80 pounds and his complexion was a deathly greenish yellow. He was upright, moral and godly—but he died. No moral or spiritual law was broken, but the dietary law was, which brings physical death even though done in ignorance. "My people are destroyed for lack of knowledge" and some "have rejected knowledge" (Hosea 4:6).

A certain research society chose three hundred Jews at random and made tests for cancer. They found not one case of cancer among these 300 Jews who observed the dietary law that God gave through Moses. In further tests, however, they found the very slight beginnings of cancer in one woman who, after she had been questioned at length, admitted that she had not kept the dietary laws with any regularity. There is not a word for cancer or its equivalent in the old pure Hebrew language. It was not known among God's ancient covenant-keeping people—"There was not one feeble person among their tribes" (Psalm 105:37).

Book Triggered by Death

The final blow that triggered the immediate writing of this book and drove the urgency of it deep into my soul was the death of a minister friend from cancer. I had not known Rev. K. long, but the bond was very close, and I so greatly valued his ministry because of its richness in the Word of God.

Rev. K. had been operated on once for cancer several years before, and was now being plagued again with its spread. I talked to him about the facts recorded in this book. He said he had been thinking along this line and had wondered if wrong eating might be the cause. He had been a big eater and lover of pork. (Incidentally, eating enormous helpings of food, especially red meats, is a bad sign. Let this be a warning signal to check yourself.)

Unfortunately his doctor was not a student of nutrition or a believer in the dietary law. He kept him on meats and sugar-loaded ice cream that actually stimulate cancer. By this time the malignancy had attacked the vital organs until there was no hope for recovery.

What a heart-wrenching tragedy to see this valuable man and his wealthy ministry come to an end. This was more than I could bear. It was the final signal to get this volume into print at the earliest possible date.

Some may retort that the work of winning souls is more important than helping people stay or get well physically or than prolonging their lives. But unless men who know the Word of God and who have the riches of experience stay well and alive physically, how can they tell the message of man's redemption? In fact the word, 'salvation,' takes in the whole man, the welfare of body, soul and spirit.

It Couldn't Happen But It Did

It cheers us to hear of hearts that are open to truth and particularly to that which blesses our lives with health, strength, and long life with its many attendant spiritual blessings. Contrariwise, it pains us to learn of those who believe themselves to be wise and yet reject God's life-saving and soul-blessing Word as the following tragic, true story reveals. It happened just prior to the fourth printing of this book early in 1976.

The man was a leading official in a long-established church and in his denomination. He was a most successful businessman, serving as the vice-president of a very large world-wide corporation. He was as financially secure as a man could be, having a lovely wife, and elegantly furnished home with all the latest electronic gadgets and appliances. His love for God and His Word was genuine, holding tenaciously to what he believed were the great truths of the Scriptures. But one thing I fear he lacked, the choicest element of Christian faith . . . humility and the resultant open heart.

There were regular monthly prayer breakfasts held at the church; he was responsible for the food that was served. Almost inevitably, some part of the swine, such as ham, would be on the menu. (Perhaps he wanted to show he had been delivered from the so-called "curse of the Law"—forgetting what Paul had written that "the Law was holy, spiritual, just and good.") A close friend of mine who attended the breakfasts was always "put on the spot" because he believed what God declared, "I am the Lord, I change not," and that His Law was given for our welfare (not salvation). This church leader 'in sympathy' for "the weaker brother" always prepared a beef-burger for my friend's breakfast.

Then the day of reckoning came. Though he was much

younger than my close friend, yet there came about a deterioration in his body. It was thought that a minor operation would correct his physical difficulty. Yet, he may have suspected something was very badly wrong. He requested that he be put into a Jewish hospital and treated by Jewish doctors. After examination, there came the terrible, shocking news that he was in the last stages of cancer. He requested that kosher meals now be given him to eat, but it was too late—he had rejected the Lord's clean diet too long.

The doctors did all in their power to save his life. They kept him alive artificially for many days. Finally, they had to break the news; they could continue this artificial life no longer. They told him, "Tomorrow morning we must take you off of this synthetic means of keeping you alive and you will be in the hands of the Lord." But my friend had reached the point of no return. When the machines were turned off, his life began to ebb until finally it flickered out. What a tragic ending and defeat to what could have been a glorious and victorious life of many more years of usefulness and happiness according to the promises of God. This was another case of God's warning: "My people are destroyed for lack of knowledge," and some "because they have rejected knowledge" (Hosea 4:6). May the Lord humble our hearts to hear, believe, obey and be blest.

With no spirit akin to "I told you so," but with a wrenched heart and mind we share this word of further warning. Our Wichita representative has just informed us (February, 1976) that a friend who ten years ago strongly ridiculed and opposed the truths we set forth in *God's Key to Health* is, at this writing, in the last stages of dying of cancer. This is not an isolated case but one in a continual pattern we have seen through the past 40 years. "The wise will hear and increase learning . . . Hear . . . and the years of thy life shall be many. They are life . . . and health to all their flesh" (Proverbs 1:5; 4:10,22).

Satan would blind men to God's truth and seek to destroy them physically and thereby hinder the work of the Most High and rob our matchless Redeemer-Messiah of the praises due to His Name. Satan hates God's law and is a past-master in getting agents to mock, ridicule, and laugh it to scorn, unto their own destruction and death.

"For in death there is no remembrance of thee: in the grave who shall give thee thanks?" (Psalm 6:5).

"The dead praise not the Lord, neither any that go down into silence" (Psalm 115:17).

"For the grave cannot praise thee, death cannot celebrate thee . . . The living, the living, he shall praise thee as I do this day. . . ." (Isaiah 38:18,19).

Our all-wise God declares of His law, "Hear, O my son, and receive my sayings; and the years of thy life shall be many" (Proverbs 4:10). In this life only, do we have the opportunity of praising our Lord in adverse circumstances and among His adversaries. All praise Him *in Heaven,* but let us seek to inspire others to praise Him *on earth,* which bears a far greater weight and can influence and even determine the destiny of immortal souls. Man's chief end is to glorify God. "Let everything that hath breath praise the Lord" (Psalm 150:6).

Without any question, the breaking of these life-preserving dictary laws of the Almighty is a cause of much cancer, as well as many other diseases. Many folk will pay hundreds of dollars to an *"earth-doctor"* for a trial diet and ignore a perfect one prescribed by *heaven's Great Physician,* "in whom are hid all the treasures of wisdom and knowledge" (Colossians 2:3). Is this the better part of wisdom?

A special bulletin in the *U.S. News and World Report* was issued March 8, 1976, under the subhead, "STRANGE AND DEADLY FLU." Following are some excerpts:

Today's Flu. In spite of more than 4,200 deaths in the present epidemic in the U.S., hog flu doesn't seem to be implicated. Another strain—A-Victoria—is the one on the rampage. As of February 27, only 11 cases of hog flu have been confirmed—all at Fort Dix. That was the first recorded outbreak caused by the virus, which since the early 1930s has been known to infect pigs and hogs. Viruses weren't discovered until the 1930s. Thus, there's only indirect evidence that the antibodies in some people lead many scientists to suspect the hog-flu strain was the culprit in 1918–19—a world-wide ravaging epidemic that took 20 million lives just after World War I.

Epidemics coming? But the hog-virus strain may surface again in the late fall or early winter, bringing with it the possibility of raging epidemics. Unfortunately, flu shots you have taken up to now provide no protection against hog flu.

On Wednesday, March 24, 1976, President Ford issued a very serious and alarming warning which we heard over CBS radio. He stated that all American citizens—men, women, youth and children—should be vaccinated against a possible outbreak of the Swine Flu by the fall, for fear of another epidemic such as took the lives of 500,000 Americans following World War I in 1918 and that killed over 20,000,000 throughout Europe and other parts of the world. (If any should suggest the unfailing Scriptural solution [Exodus 15:26] he would no doubt receive the same stock professional reply—not, "That's too simple," but the more profound and dignified—"That's an over-simplification of the prognosis." Let medical science make a study [1] of those who govern their lives according to the divine laws and precepts, [2] and those that do not. The findings would be happily staggering.)

The cost of this nation-wide inoculation program was stated to be over $135 million.

10

Peter's Vision

"What about Peter's vision on the housetop and the vessel let down from heaven with all manner of unclean beasts?" is a common query of those who believe this trance nullifies the dietary law. Read carefully Acts chapter 10. This account of God sending a Jew (Peter) for the first time to a Gentile (non-Jew) with the gospel marks the actual beginning of "the times of the Gentiles," *spiritually,* or to be more technically correct, the *beginning* of "the fullness of the Gentiles."

The Jewish Gospel

Up to this point, none of the Jews, even seven years after the day of Pentecost, believed that the gospel was for any other nation but Israel. Had you, if a Gentile, lived in Jerusalem immediately following the Pentecostal outpouring of the Spirit of God, the first century Jewish disciples would have passed you by and never attempted to tell you of Messiah's redeeming gospel.

The Jewish people knew that they were God's chosen people, and that they were to be separated unto Him. They were not to mingle socially, especially *not to EAT,* with the heathen, lest they, in process of time, be defiled nationally through intermarriage, and finally perish through assimilation (Ezra 9 and 10).

Approximately seven years after Pentecost this vision came to Peter, sending him to the house of Cornelius, the Gentile. But, though he obeyed God, still he did not know at this time "for what intent ye have sent for me." As we read in Acts 11:19, until this time they had preached "the Word to none but unto the Jews only."

Honest Questions

Let us without prejudice open our minds and search diligently for the truth God is giving us here. First, let us remember this vessel with all manner of unclean beasts came down FROM HEAVEN. The Lord did not show him a den of snakes or a hog lot ON EARTH. It is also essential that we keep in mind that the vessel was caught up again INTO HEAVEN. Now, did the words, "Rise, Peter, kill and eat," mean that God was repealing the dietary laws? Is God reversing Himself on physical hygiene and sanitation in His requirement that a clean people have clean food? Did Christ's work on the cross perform a biological miracle in these filthy animals that made their flesh harmless to eat and fit for human consumption? Did the dispensation of grace and the coming of the gospel so alter the gastric processes and digestive apparatus of man that all unclean meats will now build healthy bodies instead of producing disease and result in death as they did before?

Peter's Conclusion

Peter himself did not conclude this as we read in verse 17, since "PETER DOUBTED IN HIMSELF what this vision which he had seen should mean." There is not a shadow of an inkling, as the context clearly proves, that Peter believed this vision had anything to do with a change in the dietary law. The unclean beasts, fowls and creeping things were *symbols of the unclean pagan nations,* even as they are today. America has an unclean bird, the eagle, as an insignia and coat of arms; England has the lion; Russia, the bear; China, the dragon, etc., all of which are unclean. Peter was now being sent to the house of Cornelius, the Gentile, one of an "unclean" nation.

Under the Mosaic Covenant, God instructed the Hebrew people to consider all non-Jewish nations (Gentiles, goyim) as unclean. They were to be separated from them unto their God-given covenant. As a clean, disease-free diet would keep them strong physically as individuals so, more important, they were to keep pure socially that they might remain strong as a people, nationally.

There is not a shred of evidence that Peter's vision had anything to do with diet, apart from the fact the Lord was telling him not to hesitate to "arise and EAT" with these UN-CLEAN Gentiles, for the sake of sharing the world-inclusive Messianic message with them.

Peter's own testimony regarding the vision was, "God hath showed me that I should not call any MAN [not animal] common or unclean." Cornelius, an Italian, was of one of the nations which the Jews had considered unclean. Later, when the church officials at Jerusalem called Peter on the carpet, they contended with him and accused him of going "into men UN-CIRCUMCISED, and DID EAT with them."

Uncircumcision was a mark of uncleanness. If a man (Jewish or proselyte) was not circumcised, he was cut off from God's covenant. In the 11th chapter of Acts, Peter rehearsed the matter to the apostles, who were shocked that he would associate with one of an unclean nation. He testified that, as he spoke the Word of God, the Spirit of God from heaven fell on these "unclean," and that they experienced the same wonderful cleansing that they themselves had received. This cleansing was symbolized by Peter commanding them to be baptized in the name of the Lord.

No unprejudiced scholar, after a careful study and exegesis of this passage, can rightfully contend that here the Almighty repeals the clean, health-building dietary law and pure food ministration, and gives an across-the-board license to eat all unclean, germ-laden, disease-producing scavenger animal flesh.

Can it be, when from the beginning of time it was an abomination to even touch the carcasses of these unclean beasts lest one be contaminated with a contagious disease, that in a moment of time this same animal is made a wholesome food delicacy for human consumption? Such reasoning is unthinkable, illogical, and unscriptural.

People, Not Pigs

If we hold the view that all unclean animals were made clean and holy by reason of Peter's vision, then most assuredly *all the unclean pagan peoples* of all nations *were made clean and holy* since *the vision clearly deals with their cleansing.*

If such reasoning were carried out, then we must conclude that all missionary endeavor and the preaching of Christ's gospel is unnecessary. If Peter's trance sanctified filthy and abominable animals, it certainly sanctified the unclean pagan peoples since they are the objects of the vision.

Did this vision automatically make every unclean unbelieving pagan, including all wicked blasphemers, clean and fit for heaven, *God's habitation?* No, of course not. And neither did it make the loathsome unclean animals clean and fit for your *body* (also God's habitation), which is called "the temple of God" (I Corinthians 3:16). There had to be a real miracle work of God's transforming grace wrought in the hearts of these unclean pagans before they could be accepted into the place of God's abode. There has been no such work wrought on the flesh of unclean beasts that makes them fit for God's physical temple. The animals God spoke of are not available, for they were "caught up again *into heaven.*" Our all-wise Lord took this precaution lest we should confuse the vision with dietetics.

The Lord is dealing with *people* in the vision, not *pigs.* The animals were merely figures and types. We get into very severe trouble and error by carrying spiritual types and shadows into the literal realm. We do violence to the Scriptures and open the door to false teachings which can be very destructive.

Rightly Dividing the Word

We have an example of this in the Eucharist (Holy Communion). Jesus said, concerning the bread, "Take eat, this is my body." And again concerning the wine, "This is my blood" (Matthew 26:26–28). In John 6:53 Jesus said, "Except ye eat the flesh of the Son of Man and drink His blood ye have no life in you." Missionaries from South America tell us of churches that teach that this is literally true (as some do in America); i.e., the bread actually becomes the body of Christ and the wine actually His blood. When the communicants take the bread, and perhaps have a cold and begin to cough, they immediately put their hand up to their mouth for fear of coughing out and losing their eternal life. This superstitious fear comes from taking this passage literally.

Blasphemers, in order to ridicule, have taken this passage literally and have painted a picture of the Lord's Supper with the disciples actually chewing on the body of Jesus Christ. This is the violence we do the Scriptures and untold damage we do ourselves and others, by taking literally something which God is using as a figure and symbol to teach a blessed truth. Jesus went on to explain, "The flesh profiteth nothing. The Words that I speak unto you they are Spirit and they are life" (John

6:63). Let us be careful to "rightly divide the Word of Truth" (II Timothy 2:15).

The Apostle Peter, in his latter years, after God had showed him that he must "shortly put off this tabernacle" (body) still considered the swine unclean as he writes in his last letter, II Peter 2:22, and likens *unclean animals* to the *reprobate* and the *ungodly* when he says, "It is happened unto them according to the true proverb, The dog is turned to his own vomit again; and the sow that was washed to her wallowing in the mire."

Peter many years after his house-top vision uses the swine as a symbol of a man as low as he can picture him, in his filth and fallen state.

We need to reiterate that in this vision the vessel *came from heaven,* and was *caught up again into heaven.* Here the Lord takes every precaution to keep man from misinterpreting Peter's vision. The 'animals' cleansed were in that vessel and it's in heaven. These on earth are still unclean even as the unbelieving Gentiles that need a work of God's grace done within.

Regarding the true application, I am glad the vessel was caught up again into heaven, showing that the prayers of Cornelius, the former unclean Gentile, had come up to God. God had accepted his repentance and in return had poured out His blessed Spirit upon him and made actual the cleansing that the Redeemer purchased for him upon the cross.

Cornelius now has been accepted, and in fact has been *"caught up into heaven"* as a cleansed heathen, PRAISE THE LORD! We should rejoice that we Gentiles, unclean pagans, were moved upon by the *holy* Spirit of God, who revealed the cleansing fountain opened to the house of David and to the inhabitants of Jerusalem for sin and uncleanness, which has also been opened to us through Christ Jesus, the Messiah (Zechariah 13:1; Acts 10:34,35; 11:18).

11

Other Various Objections

Truth About Meats

Let us consider another traditional objection to the keeping of the dietary law of God. In I Timothy chapter 4, the Apostle Paul warns that the Spirit speaks expressly of those who will in the latter times depart from the faith, who will forbid to marry and command to abstain from meats, "which God hath created to be received with thanksgiving, of them which believe and know the truth." In the Greek this reads, "which God hath created for reception." It is clearly inferred that not all meats were "created to be received."

"Which believe and know the truth," about what? What truth was Paul speaking of here? We need ever to be reminded that in those days when God's people spoke of "the truth" they referred to the Scroll of the Hebrew Scriptures and the five books of Moses in particular, called the Torah. It was in this divine revelation this *truth* of the dietary law was imparted, which Paul refers to in passing, lest some might cast it aside and get into error. Why otherwise should the apostle make this insertion? Paul's *subject* was the *eating of meats,* therefore the phrase, "which believe and know the truth" about the dietary law, can be the only implication.

Creatures to Be Received

Paul continues in verse 4, "For every creature of God is good, and nothing to be refused, if it be received with thanksgiving." Those who contend for the eating of all the unclean meats make a play on words here. Some would interpret verse 4 to read, "Every creature is good, and nothing to be refused, if it be received with thanksgiving." This is doing violence to the passage. This would include every poisonous reptile, venomous serpents, deadly vipers, even to the wriggling mass of loathsome maggots and worms that feed on dead rotten carcasses. Not only so, but it would be approving cannibalism, the eating of humans. We, of course, know this is not the case.

If this be the right interpretation of this passage, one is left open to, and should not refuse, the following potential dinner:

As a starter, rattlesnake cocktail; your choice of lizard or mouse soup, angle-worm-termite-tomato combination salad, a big fat juicy rare rat roast and for those who do not relish roast rat, something lighter—like a cockroach, or black widow spider sandwich. For steak lovers, a choice rat-terrier dog or tomcat. For dessert, how about maggots and flies sundae?

You say, "That's revolting and ridiculous." No, not if "EVERY CREATURE" is good for dietary purposes as many contend. The above creatures are not one whit filthier than the swine. In fact, the hog will and does eat any and all of the said dead creatures. Can we eat this filth and expect to stay well?

What is the proper interpretation of this passage? Here is the simple logic: Paul, in using the expression, "of God," is not saying, "every creature that God has created." He is not distinguishing between those He created and those He did not create. That would be ridiculous. What other kinds of creatures are there?

By way of illustration: To contend that the statement, "Every man of God is worthy to be received into your home" means, that "Every man that God has created is worthy to be received into your home," all will agree is false. The first declaration taken at face value is true, the second is false. The same reasoning holds true when the word, "creature," is substituted for "man." Every *creature of God* is good" but not "every creature that God has created is good" for consumption as nutritious for the temple of God, your body.

To say, "every man is good," or "every creature is good" is not true. But to say "every man *of God*" or "every creature *of God* is good," is true. To say that every creature is good and not to be refused as food for your body is just as false as to say that every man is good and worthy to be received into your home. We must rightly divide the Word of truth. Ponder this carefully.

God's people distinguished between the clean and unclean, the holy and unholy, that which was "of God" and that which was not. They never held the unclean and unholy to be "of God" (Leviticus 11:44–47).

Sanctified by the Word

Some, in reading this passage totally disregard the expression, "sanctified BY THE WORD OF GOD." To contend one can sit down to a table of these bad, germ-laden, unclean things and sanctify it *by prayer* is false. The Bible does not say so. What we eat, Paul writes, first must be sanctified (set apart) "by the Word of God" (verse 5). The only accepted and written Scriptures that early Christians had was the so-called Old Testament, mainly the Torah (the law), and the prophets. This is the WORD OF GOD Paul is speaking about. There was none other so acknowledged at that time. (Later, Paul's letters and other writings were to be accepted also as divinely inspired Scripture.) The Word of God was clear in sanctifying (setting apart) certain meats for human consumption (Leviticus 11 and Deuteronomy 14). So Paul states in I Timothy 4 that the things we eat should be sanctified (set apart) "by the word of God and prayer." Certainly then we should *pray* and ask God's blessing over these things that are set apart by *the Word of God* for our tables. These sanctified meats are therefore spoken of as "of God" as Paul does in verse 4.

It would be just as ridiculous for me to try to sanctify by prayer something that was strictly prohibited in the dietary law (the Word of God) as it would be for me to attempt to sanctify by prayer some breach of the moral law (of God's Word). Some that attempt to do this eventually find it is to their own hurt and even to their sorrow and shame. However beautiful, practical and necessary we feel a new automobile may be, we cannot by prayer sanctify stealing it when the moral law of God says, "Thou shalt not steal": nor can we sanctify a dirty, filthy hog to our body's health when God states, "These shall ye not eat." Why should we destroy ourselves? Remember, the laws of God cannot be 'broken'; we merely break ourselves over them.

Body Defiled, Not Heart

Another objection to the observance of the dietary law is a passage found in St. Matthew 15:11. Some who are absolutely confident that this passage completely nullifies the dietary laws, argue, "Did not Jesus say, 'Not that which goeth into the mouth defileth a man; but that which cometh out of the mouth, this defileth a man'?" The Lord Himself explains the passage in verses 17 and 18. The same Scripture is even more clearly given in Mark 7 as Jesus relates that food (the literal translation of the word "meats" in verse 19, is "food"—he is not speaking of flesh) cannot defile the man "Because it entereth not into his heart" (Mark 7:19). Would Jesus break any part of the law or suggest such to us? It is true that breaking the dietary law does not defile the spiritual heart but it certainly can defile the human flesh. If anyone doubts that the body can be defiled because we are under grace, a dose of strychnine will quickly convince him. Medical records are replete with cases of those who have died of food poisoning. There is abundant proof that our bodies are under the same rigid laws that God made in the beginning.

Exceptions

We are told there are exceptions to all laws. We agree to this, but they are very few and should not be gambled with. Let us be very sure of our ground and cautious lest we fall into 'something over our heads.' In Mark 16:17,18, when Jesus gave 'the great commission,' He stated, "And these signs shall follow them that believe; in my Name . . . they shall take up serpents." This did not mean that Jesus made every deadly serpent harmless, nor did it mean because we believe in miracles that we should deliberately play with vipers for exhibition's sake or to display our great faith. A missionary in the line of duty who might encounter a deadly snake, could believe God for special protection and deliverance and not suffer from its deadly fangs and sting, as the Apostle Paul in his experience on the island of Melita (Acts 28:1–6).

In the same way we should not tempt God or put ourselves in jeopardy regarding our physical health by constantly consuming these prohibited meats such as swine, etc., that are filled with tiny deadly serpents. Let us not play the fool as the religious snake charmers who tempt God under the guise of demonstrating their great faith. This is not faith but presumption, which God hates.

What about exceptions, such as I Corinthians 10:27,28 where one is invited into a pagan home? In this case it was meat offered to idols and some early Christians considered it defiled by evil spirits. It is this superstition Paul is dealing with in the above passage. Only in a matter of 'life and death' and God's Name being reproached should an exception be made to the dietary law.

Read Jeremiah 35 regarding divine prohibitions in connection with the fifth commandment. There is no conflict of allegiance in God's commands.

The converted heathen should be taught to turn from this unclean practice as well as from all the other harmful and unholy customs and habits.

Read I John 2:3–6;5:2,3.

There are other exceptions as in isolated cases where missionaries must accept the hospitality of the natives who serve these unclean meat dishes. In such a case, I believe they could claim a special dispensation, and trust God to protect them from the infinitesimally small cripplers and killers. However, there are very few spots on the face of the earth where sufficient protein foods are not found without taking the risk of being poisoned. If clean animals are not available, the protein diet can be supplemented through nuts, soybeans, sunflower seeds, various grains, dairy dishes and many other such good, nutritious foods.

For illustration: I have a friend who served as a communications engineer during World War II. While stringing communication lines deep in a jungle area on a South Pacific island, he became lost. For eight months he was separated from his company and wandered around in the jungles, living only on coco-

nuts, fruit, nuts and other jungle vegetation edibles. At the close
of this long ordeal, he said he was in better health living on this
diet than he had ever been in all of his life.

We should be in a very bad situation indeed before finding
it necessary to take chances with these subtle killers that lurk
in scavenger flesh.

Responsible for the Temples of God

Call to mind: we are responsible to God as custodians of our
bodies, the temples of His Spirit. "If any man defile the temple
of God, him shall God destroy; for the temple of God is holy,
which temple ye are" (I Corinthians 3:17). Since this passage is
written to Christians about their bodies, Paul, without question,
refers to the destruction of their bodies as He does in I Corinthians 5:5, "For the destruction of the flesh." This does not always
or necessarily mean an arbitrary action on God's part, but that
a 'broken law' of God actually destroys the man. We need a
revival of an awesome positive reverential fear of the Eternal
God and His Word. "A son honoreth his father and a servant
his master; if then I be a father, where is mine honor, and if I
be a master, where is my fear? saith the Lord of hosts" (Malachi
1:6).

The Area of "Adiaphorous"

There are some who look for any loophole, legal or illegal,
to justify their "breaking" the laws of God. They would quote,
"there is nothing unclean of itself" (Romans 14:14), and "Happy
is he that condemneth not himself in the thing which he al-
loweth" (verse 22). They fail to take the context into account.
When Paul here speaks of one that "eats all things," he differen-
tiates between a vegetarian and one who eats all meats, according to the holy dietary law of God. To the true Jew—and Paul

called himself a Hebrew of the Hebrews—*all the laws of God are as firmly fixed as the law of gravity.* They would not question the dietary law one whit, any more than they would the moral law. On the premise some interpret this Scripture, we might as well conclude that Paul was encouraging the breaking of the Ten Commandments when he said four times, "All things are lawful for me" (I Corinthians 6:12 and 10:23). According to such reasoning one could murder, steal, lie, commit adultery, blaspheme God and blindly expect no punishment. This is unreasonable.

What is the apostle setting forth? It is this: The law is good and spiritual, but we, being naturally weak, were unable to keep it perfectly, and so we became lawbreakers and prisoners under its death penalty. God then, in order to be just, visited us through Jesus who kept the law perfectly; now God (in Christ) presents us with the gift of this perfect righteousness, which we receive by faith. Contrariwise, our sin was laid on him so it was mandatory for Him to die (our death . . . in our stead). "For he has made him (Christ) to be sin for us, who knew no sin; that we might be made the righteousness of God in him" (II Corinthians 5:21).

But remember, it was the transgression of God's holy law that put us in the death cell. Did our Lord leave heaven's glory, suffer the agonies of Gethsemane, die the ignominious death on a Roman cross to buy us a license to commit sin, to transgress His laws? A thousand times no. Praise God we are free, gloriously free from the law's *guilt* and *penalty.* Christ paid for all transgressions from the beginning to the end of time, "for the sins of the whole world" (I John 2:2). Regarding eternal salvation, "All things are lawful," for a penalty cannot be exacted twice. A man can die only once for sin, and Christ paid that death. But I remind you that he who receives Christ, has His Spirit infused into him (Galatians 4:6) and has His law written on his heart (Jeremiah 31:33; Hebrews 8:10). Set free, yes, not as a slave to sin, but our relationship now is that of an obedient righteous son to a Father. We want now, above all, to please Him for "the love of Christ constraineth us."

Paul here is speaking of the "adiaphorous" (Romans 14), the area on which the Scriptures do not particularly speak. In such matters, it is true, we have freedom to act and react according to the perfect law of liberty.

For instance as in certain amusements, games, and even the drinking of certain beverages: in France, Christians think nothing about drinking wine; in America, most Christians frown upon it. When the Evangelist Charles E. Finney spoke against worldly evils, he classed the use of tobacco and coffee in the same category. In the South some real true Christians use the former without condemnation, and in the North the latter is used without any compunction of conscience. To the Evangelist Finney, they were both sin. In the South, mixed swimming for years was frowned upon, while generally accepted in the North. Styles and fashions are another area spoken of in the Scriptures in general, but not in detail.

Worldly amusements may run from black to light shades of grey and nearly white. All would agree on the evil of burlesque shows while others would go so far as to say that even gospel films are wrong. Let every man be persuaded in his own mind. Our attitude in these areas should be as Paul's, "It is good neither to eat flesh, nor to drink wine, nor any thing whereby thy brother stumbleth, or is offended, or is made weak" (Romans 14:21).

The Apostle Paul writes that one man esteems one day holy above all the rest, while another man esteems all days holy, as implied in the original text. In both instances, however, the essential thing is that we do all things, "as to the Lord." The key verse of Romans 14 is the 9th, "For to this end Christ both died, and rose, and revived, that he might be LORD both of the dead and living." If we make Him LORD, we will be obedient unto His Word. If we *love Him* that gave the law we will desire above all to be obedient to it.

> His law is my delight,
> His will I now obey, and
> all the while I'm singing,
> "glory."

12

Jesus Versus Swine

Jesus' Attitude Toward Dietary Law

What was Jesus' attitude toward God's holy dietary law? First, we know He observed the law or He could not have been the world's Redeemer. He had to fulfill all the divine requirements of the law completely in order to be the perfect sacrifice, without the least condemnation, sin or guilt. There is never a record where He ate anything unclean or violated the healthful and nutritional laws of God; if He had, He could not have faced the throng with the query, "Which of you convinceth me of transgression?"

Jesus and the Man of Gadara

In three of the Gospels, we have the story of Jesus crossing the Sea of Galilee and coming to the country of the Gadarenes. As He came ashore, a man met Him who was possessed by demons, exceeding fierce and could not be chained or tamed by any man, and who was naked and dwelt among the tombs. Jesus commanded these unclean spirits to come out of the man and He sent them into a herd of swine feeding nearby. The herd immediately ran violently down a steep place into the sea and perished. Mark tells us there were about 2,000 that choked in the sea.

Jesus, during His life and ministry, proved Himself a conservationist. He did not believe in destroying anything good and useful. When He fed the five thousand (men), a crowd that could have numbered into the scores of thousands when counting the women and children, He told His disciples to gather up the fragments (small broken pieces) that nothing be lost. It was quite a chore to gather up all the pieces of bread, and yet He destroyed 2,000 swine with one stroke. Jesus would not have destroyed them had they been good for human nourishment. He could have dispensed of these evil spirits in other ways as He did at other times when He cast them out.

The reaction of the people in Jesus' day to His destroying the swine is an interesting commentary on human nature of this and every generation. It brought about a revolution: "The whole city [not just the owners] came out—and besought him to depart out of their coasts" (Matthew 8:34). They preferred to see a man insane and torn by wild demons, risking the danger of the havoc he might cause them or their children, rather than have this loathsome swine delicacy taken from their tables. (Evidence that most in this area were not Jews.) They would rather have their hogs than the true prophet of God (Deuteronomy 18:15–19). In fact, they rejected Him and prayed Him to leave their country since He destroyed their pork supply.

Human nature hasn't changed, therefore, we should not be surprised when someone furiously or with an adroit superior air, contends for a scavenger diet. If this was the human reaction to Jesus' stand on this question, is it surprising that there is a similar emotional response today? "The servant is not above his Lord." Let us be content to know the truth and be free of "all these evil diseases" (Deuteronomy 7:15), and be thankful for a God who has clearly marked the way to vibrant health and strength.

Jesus and the Prodigal Son

Read the story of the prodigal son in St. Luke's Gospel, chapter 15:11–32. Our Lord in giving us this account, in order to describe the lowest depths to which the prodigal had fallen, depicted him feeding on the husks that the SWINE ate. On the return of the prodigal to his home, how did his father celebrate? Did he say, "Bring hither the fatted hog and kill it and let us eat and be merry?" No, it was "the fatted CALF," a clean animal. I would choose to follow our Lord in example and precept in such matters, rather than join our modern "money changers"—or rather—"diet changers" and their parade to the hospital which could have been avoided. (Hospitals, of course, are a great boon and blessing to many. Room and beds should be left to those whose suffering stems from other causes than wrong dietetics.)

Jesus and the Law

In Matthew 5:17–19, Jesus said, "Think not that I am come to destroy the law or the prophets. I am not come to destroy but to fulfill. For verily I say unto you, Till heaven and earth pass, one jot or one tittle shall in no wise pass from the law, till all be fulfilled. Whosoever, therefore, shall break one of these least commandments, and shall teach men so, he shall be called the least in the kingdom of heaven: but whosoever shall do and teach them, the same shall be called great in the kingdom of heaven." (We will deal more fully with this subject in the following chapter.)

Can you sing, "I would be like Jesus" and mean it unless you accept His attitude toward God's holy, joy-generating, life-preserving law? Give this nutritional cleanliness your thoughtful and prayerful attention.

13

The Old Testament
As Related to the New

How are the 'Old' Testament and the law related to the Christian and the 'New' Testament? What position did Jesus, the apostles and the early church take on this question? It is very important that we rightly settle this in our minds in order to keep ourselves from error, frustration and even serious trouble and heartache.

Each the Other's Counterpart

The Bible is a TWO-edged sword with both the so-called Old and the New Testaments essential to spiritual warfare.

The Old Testament is God's truth enfolded—in the New it is unfolded to the nations. In the Old Testament, events are predicted—in the New they are (or ultimately will be) fulfilled. In the Old, Messiah is concealed—in the New He is revealed. The Old is the root—the New is the branch. The Old is the bud —the New is the flower. The New Testament is impossible without the Old, as impossible as leaves and fruit without the branch and tree. One is the counterpart of the other, both are incomplete without the other.

The true Messiah of the New Testament is the Jehovah of the Old, incarnate. In the burning bush God said to Moses, "Say . . . the 'I AM' hath sent me unto you." Jesus said, "Before

Abraham was, I AM." This is His Name—not I was, or shall be, but the great "I AM." Christ is the personification, the express image of God (Hebrews 1:1–3). God revealed Himself through the spoken Word on Mount Sinai in the Old Testament and in the incarnate (in flesh), living Word on Mount Calvary in the New (John 1:1–3; Luke 23:33–38; Revelation 19:11–13).

We have referred in a previous chapter to Jesus' concept of the old sacred Scriptures as recorded in Matthew 5:17–19. Jesus said He "came not to destroy the law . . . but to fulfill" that it might be fulfilled in us who believe on Him. Instead of minimizing the law, Jesus actually magnified the law as revealed in this passage (Matthew 5). He fulfilled all the law perfectly or He could not have been the transgressor's substitute and sin offering (Isaiah 53).

Why Golgotha? Calvary? It was *our violation* of these COMMANDMENTS that temporarily blotted out the "Sun of Righteousness" (Malachi 4:2) from heaven; that sent Him to a dark Gethsemane, symbolized by the three hours of "darkness over all the earth" at His crucifixion (Luke 23:44–45). He hung between heaven and earth as forsaken of God and man, to pay the death penalty for our transgression, dying the death of a hated criminal. His very soul was poured out as our sin-offering (Isaiah 53:11,12). Dare we imply by lip or life that He did this that we might transgress the laws of the Moral Governor of the Universe with impunity? On the contrary; this, the greatest event of all history, was displaying God's evaluation of the law to the whole world, showing the awful penalty of its transgression, and the tremendous price of man's redemption. The cross made sin (transgression) become exceeding sinful, and should drive us to yield ourselves unto God, "that the righteousness of the law might be fulfilled in us, who walk not after the flesh but after the Spirit" (Romans 8:4).

We took note in another passage of Paul's esteem of the law

of God where he reminds us that ordinances are not the most important "but the keeping of the commandments of God" (I Corinthians 7:19). And in Romans 7:12 and 14 he tells us the law is holy, just, good and spiritual. It is for our benefit and blessing.

Paul, before Felix, declared:

"This I confess unto thee that after the way which they call heresy, so worship I the God of my fathers BELIEVING ALL THINGS WHICH ARE WRITTEN IN THE LAW and in the prophets" (Acts 24:14).

Paul writes in Romans 7:22 as King David did,

"I delight in the law of God" [for] "the love of Christ constraineth me" (II Corinthians 5:14).

In the book of Hebrews, the Apostle declares what the new covenant (New Testament) really is, and he quotes from the prophet Jeremiah (31:31–34) where our Lord proclaims,

"This is the covenant that I will make with the house of Israel after those days, saith the Lord; I will put my law into their minds and write them in their hearts. . . ." (Hebrews 8:10).

The Apostle John speaks to us in this regard:

"And hereby we know that we know him if we keep his commandments. He that saith 'I know him' and keepeth not his commandments is a liar and the truth is not in him" (I John 2:3,4). And again, "And whatsoever we ask we receive of him because we keep his commandments and do those things that are pleasing in his sight" (I John 3:22).

"By this we know that we love the children of God when we love God and keep his commandments. For this is the love of God that we keep his commandments and his commandments are not grievous" (I John 5:2,3).

First Christians and Apostles Honored Law

When first century Christians gathered at the Temple in Jerusalem, or in the synagogues, they read from the old Hebrew Scriptures, primarily the Torah (first five books). This is the Scripture they used at all their meetings and rehearsed in all their devotions. When they used the word "Scriptures," they referred to the so-called Old Testament. Now with the first coming of the Messiah, God was beginning to form the other edge of this two-edged sword, with Christ (Messiah) in them by God's Spirit, that was to make His truth doubly effective in the world in destroying evil and sending laborers to gather the spiritual harvest.

Final Conclusion of Early Church

At the church council in Jerusalem (Acts 15) the apostles were very careful to make it clear that they were not saved by keeping the law. Some were trying to make the law a yoke and a burden, as a prerequisite of and essential to redemption. We need constantly to be reminded that we can never earn Heaven by our works. It is a gift. This, Christ purchased for us at Calvary, through offering His sinless life as a sacrifice for our transgressions. When one receives Christ (John 1:12) as sin-atoning Saviour by simple faith, an actual miracle transaction takes place in the heart that Jesus called the new birth (John 3:1–18). We then find an entirely new set of desires occupying our hearts, a wonderful love for God's Word, God's people, God's house and a compassion for those who are "out of the way." It is Christ's Spirit that has made us new creatures as Paul states (II Corinthians 5:17). Our life is transformed because Christ gives a hatred for sin: we now see it as a destroyer. We have an intense love for righteousness because it blesses and honors God for Whom we have been created.

In a special letter to the Gentiles, the apostles sought to clarify some wrong conceptions. The letter dealt in particular with a controversy that was threatening the unity of the church. Some uninstructed Gentile converts were seeking to hold on to some of their pagan religious customs regarding meats being offered to idols and acts of fornication which had been commonly accepted in their former heathen religious practices. Some zealous Jewish believers wanted to straighten them out in a hurry and contended it was necessary to keep the law of Moses in order to be saved (Acts 15:1,2). The church council sat in session to consider this problem.

Because other points in the moral and dietary law, such as loving God, taking God's name in vain, murder, stealing, etc., as well as eating unclean meats were omitted, did not mean the apostles were here sanctioning their violation. It was taken for granted that God's whole law, moral and dietary, governing all of life, was the very foundation of Christian society.

The apostles wanted it made clear that the law could never take them to heaven, because their obedience to it could never be perfect. For this reason Christ came and became the transgressors' perfect substitute by keeping the whole law perfectly for them. This perfection is charged to the account of all those who believe on Christ, the Messiah. Hallelujah!

The letter, in part, reads, "that ye abstain from meats offered to idols, and from blood and from things strangled and from fornication, which if ye keep yourselves ye shall do well. Fare ye well" (Acts 15:29). And the final word, "We believe that through the grace [unmerited favor] of the Lord Jesus Christ we shall be saved even as they" (Acts 15:11).

What should be our conclusion in the matter? Primarily, that we are not saved by keeping any of the law, moral, dietary or ceremonial—the transgression of which was death. Christ who kept the law perfectly for us, took our transgression upon Himself and died in our place, exchanging our sins for His perfect righteousness. Because He has imparted His Spirit to us, written His law upon our hearts, we out of gratitude and love to Him should seek to follow and imitate His flawless life every moment of all our remaining days by yielding ourselves to Him that He might work "in you both to will and to do of his good pleasure" (Philippians 2:13).

14

Eating of Blood

Faith in God Threatened

In my early teens, my mother told me a story that, unbeknown to her, threatened my faith in God. To say the least, it caused me to entertain doubts about Him being a good God. She related how my grandmother in Sweden had had a terrible fear of cancer, and prayed all of her life that she would not die of this dreaded disease. However, in her latter years, it was discovered that she did have cancer and finally died as its victim. This made a terrible impression upon my mind.

Mother, who was a godly and precious saint of God, sought constantly to inspire faith in our hearts, but unwittingly this time dropped a seed that began to germinate unbelief. I reasoned, "If a godly soul such as my sainted grandmother could not have one prayer answered that she prayed all her life long, how could I dare to think that I would ever receive any special mercies at the hand of the Lord? What was the use of my trying to have faith in God?" I was so aware of all my failings and possessed a full-fledged inferiority complex. At that time, I did not know that the basis of getting audience with God and having prayers answered (for me, a pagan) was faith in Christ, His righteousness, not mine. So my reasoning tore a tremendous gouge of doubt in my soul (as much reasoning will do, unless we have sufficient knowledge of the subject).

Law Established Faith

It was not until I understood the truths set forth in this book that this matter was cleared up, i.e., that the entire universe operates according to law. I reiterate that these laws govern all of life, in every sphere and on every level. As we observe them, we will get beneficial results. If we disregard them, we will suffer evil consequences. We need constantly to remember, *For every effect there is a cause.*

As I began to analyze grandmother's dilemma in the light of these laws, the answer suddenly flashed across my mind. I recalled as a boy when mother had told me stories of her childhood, how, when it was time to butcher hogs, she was instructed to hold a bucket and catch the blood of the beast, which they saved for the purpose of making blood sausage. "This," she added, "was a real delicacy in Sweden." Now all the pieces of the puzzle fell into place. It was crystal clear that the suffering and untimely death of my grandmother was due to the transgression of the dietary law. ALL BLOOD, even of clean animals, was strictly forbidden for dietetic purposes. In the case of mother's story, it was the blood of *unclean animals,* a double offense, that triggered the sickness and death. Later, I carefully studied these Biblical laws regarding the prevention and cure of sickness and disease.

"Eat Not Blood" Scriptures

The following message comes from the World's Capital, the Seat of the Universe, Heaven:

"ONLY BE SURE that thou EAT NOT THE BLOOD: for the blood is the life; and thou mayest not eat the life with the flesh. THOU SHALT NOT EAT IT; thou shalt pour it upon the earth as water. THOU SHALT NOT EAT IT that it may go well with thee, and with thy children after thee, when thou shalt do that which is right in the sight of the Lord" (Deuteronomy 12:23–25). Here was a strict prohibition from the Almighty, regarding the eating of blood.

There are many other such passages in the Scriptures, such as is found in I Samuel 14:32–35. Under King Saul's reign, the people flew on the spoil and killed animals contrary to God's blood-letting plan, and ate the meat with the blood in it. This was a sin against the Lord because they disregarded His warning Word.

"Moreover ye shall eat no manner of blood, whether it be of fowl or of beast, in any of your dwellings.

"Whatsoever soul it be that eateth any manner of blood, even that soul shall be cut off from his people" (Leviticus 7:26,27). This actually happens, physically, when these health measures are disregarded.

"And whatsoever man there be of the house of Israel, or of the strangers that sojourn among you, that eateth any manner of blood; I will even set my face against that soul that eateth blood, and will cut him off from among his people [i.e., he will die].

"For the life of the flesh is in the blood: and I have given it to you upon the altar to make an atonement for your souls: for it is the blood that maketh an atonement for the soul.

"Therefore I said unto the children of Israel, No soul of you shall eat blood, neither shall any stranger that sojourneth among you eat blood.

"And whatsoever man there be of the children of Israel, or of the strangers that sojourn among you, which hunteth and catcheth any beast or fowl that may be eaten; he shall even pour out the blood thereof, and cover it with dust.

"For it is the life of all flesh; the blood of it is for the life thereof; therefore I said unto the children of Israel, Ye shall eat the blood of no manner of flesh: for the life of all flesh is the blood thereof: whosoever eateth it shall be cut off [physically]" (Leviticus 17:10–14).

"Only be sure that thou EAT NOT THE BLOOD: for the blood is the life; and thou mayest not eat the life with the flesh" (Deuteronomy 12:23).

Disease First in Blood

Since "the life of the flesh is in the blood," it therefore follows that any disease in the animal must first defile the blood before it can be carried into the flesh of the animal. All disease is largely blood poison incipiently. The blood picks up whatever is in the stomach, be it nutritious or poisonous, and disseminates it to the various parts of the body.

Why does a funeral director go after the corpse as soon as possible upon death? He knows that putrefaction (decay) will set in much faster with the blood left in the veins. His first job is to drain out this dead, putrid blood and inject embalming fluid. After this operation, the body can be kept an indefinite period. But even the expert embalmers of Egypt, who have been known to preserve bodies for several thousand years, could not keep a corpse from rotting without draining the dead blood. Take it from the Lord who created the body—blood is not clean, healthful food.

God had given strict instructions on the manner of killing animals. The throat was to be cut so that the heart would pump out the blood, draining it thoroughly from the flesh. This is why even in the New Testament (Acts 15:29), the apostles warned the Gentile Christians, "Abstain from blood and from things strangled." Much meat that Gentiles eat today is affected in this way, as though it were strangled, leaving the blood in the flesh, even though the animals may be listed as clean. Sheep, as a rule, are killed properly, by slitting the throat, so that most lamb is clean to eat according to the Scriptures. However, most cattle are killed today either by electricity or by a blow on the head. After the heart stops, some blood drains out, but much is left in the animal. This makes the meat weigh more and 'taste better' (?). Therefore, much of our meat today is far too bloody which, to say the least, does not contribute to one's health and may be a contributing cause of cancer and other diseases.

This is one reason our Jewish friends today demand Kosher meats that are killed according to the Scriptural plan. (Kosher means "clean, fit proper." The emblem ⓤ designates products as being Kosher—even soap made from clean animals.) Kosher meat is more free from disease than most public market meat. Make your own experiment in this matter and see how much "lighter" you feel after eating Kosher meat. For years, we have disregarded these dietetic laws of God; is it any wonder our hospitals are filled and that there are so many ailments for which doctors cannot find a special cause?

You may feel Kosher meat is too expensive as a regular diet. In this case, soak ordinary meat in water half an hour, drain, salt heavily and let set for one hour. This will draw out much of the blood.

Afterward wash and prepare as usual.

If you are not well, cut down or cut out red meats and use more fish (salmon, tuna, perch, bass, pike, etc.), chicken, nut dishes, cheese (wisely) and eggs. And remember it is false economy to think you save by buying "cheap" or unsafe foods that many times put you in doctors' offices, and in the hospital. (But chew all foods well—do not wash down with drinks. If you insist on drinking with the meal, sip it slowly.)

In the summer of 1962, the American public was informed

that certain meat packing plants were "tenderizing beef on the hoof." Ten minutes before the steer is to be slaughtered, technicians inject "papain" into the veins. Think of it; in ten minutes, this powerful injection so thoroughly innoculates the entire huge animal's body, and so affects every tissue, that when the meat is cooked, the tissues are so broken down, "tenderized," that steaks and roasts "melt in your mouth."

Someone has asked, "If papain can 'tenderize' the great hulk of an entire beef carcass in ten minutes, what will it do to my stomach and to my system?" We may well ask this. We are, of course, told on absolute authority that "there is no risk." Can we depend on that? (Incidentally one million steers were papainized the first year.)

Here is a household hint from *The Wichita Eagle* that gives you a pretty good idea how powerful this stuff is! "Remove blood stains from fabric with meat tenderizer. Cover stain with tenderizer; apply warm water to make a paste. After 15 to 30 minutes, sponge with cold water. Launder as usual."

A Solemn Sex Warning:

There is no doubt that much sex perversion and sex excesses that have led to tragedy and death have their roots in the disregard of this law. When the blood of beasts are taken into the human body, they create and stimulate animal passions beyond man's control. When we observe God's law, we will find a God-given control adequate to keep these normal procreative powers in check according to His divine plan and purpose.

So much more could be said on the subject of blood, but it is sufficient that God has prohibited it. Shall we obey God or man? Upon whose word shall we risk our health, our strength and our very lives?

15

Eating of Fat

Forbidden by God

"It shall be a perpetual statute for your generations throughout all your dwellings that ye eat NEITHER FAT nor blood" (Leviticus 3:17).

So much has been said and currently written on this subject, it is superfluous to add anything further. It can be conservatively stated that excess fat intake has been found by the best authorities to be a killer.

Bible and Science Agree

The University of California issued one of the first bulletins I have read on this subject, which corroborated the dietary law that God gave to Moses over fourteen hundred years before Christ. The bulletin described how the fatty protein molecules travel in the blood stream, and are deposited on the inner wall of the coronary artery. The proteins and fats are burned off, and the cholesterol is left behind. As it piles up, it narrows and irritates the artery, encouraging more formation of such deposits. It isn't long before the blood does not have sufficient room to flow freely through the veins and capillaries, and therefore, a high blood pressure condition is created which often results in a heart attack, cerebral hemorrhage, a stroke, etc. This story is being told over and over in true life every day. *Consider.*

Proven by Experience

While pastoring at Leavenworth, Kansas, I visited a middle-aged couple who had both suffered strokes. The lady, much overweight, became paralyzed and blind. I realized, after some study, that faulty nutrition was the cause of her grave condition. Their animal fat intake was at a dangerously high level. She made no attempt to correct this dietetic evil and died shortly afterward. A neighbor then came in to help take care of the man, who was paralyzed completely on one side. The neighbor had knowledge of the importance of right eating. The paralytic was taken completely off all animal fats, and given nothing but fresh vegetables, grains, nuts, fruits, etc.

Because of other commitments, it was a matter of several months before I could get back to see him. When I did, the man, who I thought would be dead or at least sick in bed, was out hoeing and working in the garden. He made a complete recovery in a relatively short time. He bent over backward in obeying the Scriptural injunction, "eat neither FAT nor blood," and fully regained his health.

SPECIAL NOTE:

It is a miracle there are not more strokes and heart attacks the way Americans overload their blood streams with fats through bacon, sausage, french fries, rich pastries, etc., not to mention ice cream, excessive butter and syrupy drinks. The blood, instead of having the texture of fine lubricating oil, is more like a thick honey. The heart and blood then begin to cry out in thirst for water to thin down this heavy blood and take some load off the heart.

Recently a friend of mine had a severe heart attack. The doctor told him his blood was far too thick; it was like trying to pump sludge through a small water pipe. Something has to give, and it will be the pump's motor. This also happens in the human body. We pour such rich heavy foods into our systems till something must give. What is it? Our motor pump, the heart. Remember our blood is soluble with water; drink plenty of it . . . between meals. What do most Americans do when their system cries out for pure water to thin down their "syrupy" blood? They get a bottle of pop or some other sweet drink, loaded with more sugar, and pour that into their blood stream. It relieves the thirst temporarily, but as soon as the sugar enters the blood stream, it thickens it more and soon they must have another drink. The blood gets rid of what it can by depositing it throughout the body in layers of fat, and so the vicious cycle continues. The more fat, the more blood vessels have to be built, the more blood manufactured to feed these extra layers, the greater load is put on an over-worked heart. The human heart can take a lot of punishment, but it has a limit. Finally, it goes on a "strike," and the man dies.

Give your body a break; drink good, fresh, clean water BE-TWEEN MEALS and see how much better you feel. (Do not dilute stomach gastric juices, by washing food down with any kind of drink.)

Fat, No. 1 Enemy of Heart

Keep in mind, that the more deposits of fat there are on a body, the more difficult is the job of the heart to pump blood to all these fatty areas. Life insurance statistics taken through the years reveal your life span is definitely short-ened through overweight. The heart is a magnificent, preci-sion-built and strong instrument, but it has its limitations, and it finally reaches the place of no return.

Regardless how sturdy and finely engineered the best auto-mobile engine may be, if you keep mixing sand and gravel with the motor oil, it will soon break down. The same principle is involved in our bodies. Need we further scientific proof? Is it not sufficient to accept the Word of God on this subject?

Here is a Scriptural illustration: One of the heinous sins of the priest sons of Eli was, that as the sacrifice was seething and before the fat was burned, according to the Scriptures, they would come and take the flesh out of the pan. They were told, "Let them not fail to BURN THE FAT presently, and THEN TAKE as much as thy soul desireth. Then he would answer him, 'Nay, but thou shalt give it to me now, if not, I will take it by force.' Wherefore the sin of the young men was very great before the Lord, for men abhorred the offering of the Lord" (I Samuel 2:12–17). It is to our peril if we plunge headlong past the Almighty's warning signs, "STOP, Danger ahead—bridge out" etc. In such cases, 'Better be safe than sorry' is no mere pleasan-try.

The Lord rebuked Eli, the priest, regarding his two sons as we read in I Samuel 2:29–31, "Who honorest thy sons above me, to make yourselves FAT with the chiefest of all the offerings of Israel, my people . . . but them that honor me, I will honor, and they that despise me, shall be lightly esteemed." Eli's fat was actually instrumental in his death, as we read in I Samuel 4:12–22. "Eli fell from off the seat backward . . . and brake his neck, and he was an old man AND HEAVY."

Let's abide by the Word of the World's Top Nutritional Authority, the Lord God Himself, "It shall be a perpetual [never ceasing] statute that ye eat NEITHER FAT nor blood."

(Incidentally, because fat is not found in rolls around your body, does not necessarily mean it is not collecting inside your blood vessels and capillaries.)

I recall a sad case: I visited a man who had just had his left leg amputated a fraction below the hip joint because of hardening of the arteries. He was not aware that through the years he had disregarded the Scriptural injunction, "to eat neither fat nor blood." As a result, these fatty globules had deposited themselves on the inside of his veins until this life stream of blood could not press through the veins to nourish the flesh, and so his leg actually withered and died. When I visited him, he showed me his right leg which looked more like a skeleton than a human limb. He was to be taken to the hospital the next day for its amputation also. It had to be cut off as near the body as possible since the blood vessels were so filled with fat and cholesterol that there was not sufficient blood to carry on the healing process of the wound any lower down. My heart wrenched within me as I saw this suffering, fulfilling the Scriptural warning that so many ignore and are "destroyed for lack of knowledge," and others "because, they reject knowledge."

Too Much and Too Late

Another case of the saddest words of tongue or pen are these: *"Too late—it might have been."* In Wichita, Kansas, we visited a man in the Veterans' Hospital whose first complaint to us was, "All they give me is this lean meat. I'll be glad when I can go home and have my favorite fat meat again." But he was going home less both of his legs which had to be amputated because the blood vessels were so filled with fatty globules and the blood could not flow through them to carry on its life-giving processes.

While we were living in Florida, another similar case was reported in which an arm and both legs of a man had to be amputated. The wife was also sick in the hospital. He said if his wife died, upon whom he was so dependent, he would commit suicide: What needless tragedies by disregarding God's directives!

Why will some, because of prejudice, try to bolster some tottering pet theory and reject these unalterable truths that could bless them with health and long life? May the Lord open all our hearts to receive all of His truth for our welfare and His glory.

We take it for granted that it is common knowledge that too much salt is damaging to the health and is a definite cause of hardening of the arteries. Soak a piece of cloth in salt water and let dry and see what can happen inside the blood vessels. Salt also causes the body to retain its liquids causing dangerous overweight. There is a temptation to use too much of it, since it highly sharpens flavors. Use it sparsely and wisely.

Though we may not always understand the many intrinsic biological or scientific aspects of dietetics, yet let us humbly accept the directives of the Word of God.

16

Divine Healing

Does Jesus Heal Today?

"Do you believe in divine healing?" is a question frequently asked, especially of those who are ailing. Let us ask, "Do we believe in the authority of Jesus Christ? Do we believe in the divine inspiration of the Holy Scriptures, which declare, 'Jesus Christ the same yesterday, today and forever' (Hebrews 13:8)?" During His earthly life He healed all that came to Him in simple faith. Do I believe, now, after He has conquered Satan at Calvary, has the keys of death and hell and has arisen victoriously over the grave, that He still can and will heal? Yes, I believe.

Why should we think that His power is limited now, and His ministry diminished? His sin-atoning death on the cross, His triumphant resurrection and ascension are the very seat and evidences of His authority. We have greater cause and grounds for faith today than those to whom the Lord ministered during His three and a half pre-resurrection years. Now He declares, "All power is given unto me in Heaven and on earth." Let this suffice.

At Capernaum, Israel, one summer day when Jesus was visiting in the home of Peter, He found Peter's mother-in-law sick in bed with a fever. When Jesus touched her hand the fever vanished, and she got out of bed and prepared dinner for them. The news of her healing soon travelled over the whole town. That evening, throngs of folk came bringing their sick and afflicted, and the divinely inspired Scriptures relate that "He cast out the [evil] spirits with His Word, and healed all that were sick . . . that it might be fulfilled which was spoken by Isaias the prophet saying, Himself took our infirmities and bare our sicknesses." Matthew quotes this Old Testament prophetic passage in relation to the physical healing ministry of Jesus (Matthew 8:14–17).

It was Jesus who said, in giving the great commission to be carried out after His departure, "And these signs shall follow them that believe—In my Name they shall lay hands on the sick and they shall recover" (Mark 16:17,18). The book of Acts abounds with evidence that Jesus did not discontinue His healing ministry after His death and resurrection, but rather continued it in and through His disciples. The Apostle James gives us instructions about anointing the sick with oil and declares, "The prayer of faith shall save the sick, and the Lord shall raise them up" (James 5:14,15—written "to the twelve tribes which are scattered broad").

Let us praise God for the faith-inspired hope that the Scriptures hold out for the sick and suffering, through Christ, the Great Physician. Some, by His divine touch, "began to amend from that hour," and to others He gave faith for on-the-spot instantaneous MIRACLE HEALING, "made every whit whole" by the resurrection power of Christ. In any case, He is to be praised, even though He may withhold healing; He has always an all-wise design for our good and God's glory.

Paul on Divine Healing

Though some seek to nullify a present-day application of the book of Acts by calling it transitional, the weight of evidence, personal experience and testimony, belies such a position. There is further evidence in other New Testament writings. The Apostle Paul addressed the First Corinthian letter to, "ALL that in EVERY PLACE call upon the name of Jesus Christ our Lord"—that takes in present-day believers. In chapter twelve, Paul gives instructions regarding the ministry of the nine gifts of the Spirit, including the "gifts of healing" as well as the "working of miracles." Read this passage.

Why should one be so audacious as to limit God's mighty power, or why should God limit Himself in this dispensation, when He has performed "miracles, signs and wonders" in every other? The skeptic cries, "Show me a miracle," but he will never see one. Jesus said, "These signs shall follow them THAT BELIEVE," not those who doubt or disbelieve. The unbeliever will attempt to "explain away" the greatest miracle. Paul declares, "What if some did not believe? Shall their unbelief make the faith of God without effect? God forbid: yea, let God be true, but every man a liar" (Romans 3:3,4; read also Acts 14:8–18; 16:16–18; 19:11,12; Romans 15:18,19).

A minister who did not believe in divine healing said to a friend of mine, "If you believe in divine healing, why don't you go to the hospital and heal all the sick?" He answered, "If you believe in salvation, why don't you go to the slums and redeem all the derelicts?" There must be a personal faith. Jesus said, "According to your FAITH, be it unto you." Blessed is the man to whom God gives faith, both for salvation and divine healing.

Reproach On Divine Healing

However, great reproach is brought upon His Name and healing ministry, when after a wonderful deliverance, the former victim forgets the Lord's command, to "Go and sin no more, lest a worse thing come upon thee." This does not necessarily mean falling into deep gross immoral sin (though it can) but most assuredly means sinning against the body, as we have set forth in other chapters of this volume.

We cannot eat like pigs, be lazy as hogs, and project a pious attitude of superior faith and claim, "the Lord is my healer." Obedience to the Word of our God is our first responsibility. "Hath the Lord as great delight in burnt offerings and sacrifices, as in obeying the voice of the Lord? Behold to obey, is better than sacrifice, and to hearken, than the fat of rams" (I Samuel 15:22).

Gluttony

Several years ago I attended a meeting where a man testified to a miraculous healing he had experienced, which at first, caused real rejoicing in my soul. He said he had had cancer of the stomach and had been unable to keep any food down, until he despaired for his life. The doctors had given him up. Then he went on to relate how he had been healed and to prove it he stated, "For my first meal I ate seven pork chops, three helpings of potatoes with gravy, three big ears of corn, two helpings of peas, four pieces of bread, three cups of coffee and two pieces of cherry pie." The Lord catalogs the glutton with the drunkard —"The drunkard and the glutton shall come to poverty" (Proverbs 23:21). Are we to be surprised if "a worse thing comes upon" such who receive healing and refuse to "sin no more"? This man needs Solomon's warning when he said, "You put a knife to your throat if you be a man given to appetite" (Hebrew

—Proverbs 23:2). He is doing it literally. I have known of some who have drunk themselves to death and there are many others who have eaten themselves to death. Thousands dig their grave with their teeth and commit suicide with a fork. It's no joke that this is a primary reason hospitals (and cemeteries) are over-populated.

Young wives that jeopardize their marriages by gluttony and laziness, which reveals itself in rolls of fat and all sorts of self-indulgence, should be warned about driving their husbands into the arms of a "like sample" that they exhibited to their husbands before the wedding day. Such destroy their marriage and themselves. Preserve both.

Neglect

Others who may not sin against their bodies in this way, may do so by mere neglect after they have experienced divine heal-ing. They seem to think God will now suspend all natural laws and automatically enforce perfect health on them. Can one who is self-indulgent, gluttonous and lazy, expect the same reward of physical fitness as one who uses discipline in all things, and as the Apostle Paul relates, "I keep my body under and bring it into subjection"? God will not pamper indulgence and dissi-pation. God does not show partiality and He is no respecter of persons.

A beautiful church edifice can be destroyed by neglecting to fortify it by paint and repair from time to time, as well as by hacking away with a pick and crowbar. The temple of our bodies can likewise be destroyed, by neglecting to fortify it by common sense health measures and with *proper food,* according to God's Word.

Divine-Natural Healing Note:

As it is expected of 'decent persons' to take baths and wash themselves regularly though they cannot be perfectly clean 100% of the time, *even so,* the Almighty expects His creatures to keep His commandments as much as humanly possible though they fall short of absolute perfection.

God said to Abraham, "I am the Almighty God [all sufficient one], walk before me and be thou perfect [of heart]" (Genesis 17:1).

Jesus said, "Be ye perfect even as your father in heaven is perfect" (Matthew 5:48).

Aspiring parents continue to hold moral perfection as a goal for the lives of their children . . . yet children many times disappoint them.

So the Almighty being holy and also just, who cannot compromise or look upon transgression with the least favor, must demand perfect righteousness and therefore provided it for us in the love-gift of Christ. And having received Him, we are enjoined to "WALK EVEN AS HE WALKED." However, knowing our imperfection, it is assuring to know that these conditional promises of healing such as Exodus 15:26 can be claimed in Christ's fulfillment of them. "For all the promises of God in Him [Christ] are yea, and in Him, Amen, unto the glory of God by us" (II Corinthians 1:20). Hallelujah! It is our blessed Lord alone Who can deliver from every moral and spiritual 'inferiority complex' and freely give us the blessing we seek. "For He is made unto us [deposited to our account] wisdom, righteousness, sanctification, and redemption: that according as it is written, He that glorieth, let him glory in the Lord" (I Corinthians 1:30,31). Amen.

Ministry of Doctors

We need to keep in mind, that according to the Biblical record, all those whom Jesus healed were what we call "hopeless cases." They were beyond the help of earthly physicians. Without question, there are many doctors who have a divine calling as much as ministers of the gospel. (However, we need also to remember that as ministers of the gospel are imperfect and fallible, so are physicians and surgeons.) God has used doctors to alleviate much pain and suffering, and to aid in restoring sick bodies. What a great blessing is such a simple thing as the irrigation of an ear that is stopped and deafened by wax and foreign matter, the cleansing of a wound, and the setting of broken bones, etc., as well as more intricate means of therapy. Let us thank God for those true doctors whose first concern is to help suffering humanity, to minister to the living, not just to make a living. Luke was a physician who travelled much with Paul and who perhaps first gave him the advice that Paul passed on to Timothy, "Drink no longer water but use a little wine for thy stomach's sake and thine often infirmities" (I Timothy 5:23). There are many simple remedies that we should not feel too "spiritually big" to use because we believe in divine healing. It was God that healed King Hezekiah, though the prophet Isaiah told him to apply a poultice of figs, according to the Word of the Lord (II Kings 20; Isaiah 38). Let us be as practical, and miracle-believing, as the Word of God.

17

Natural Healing

"I am the Lord that healeth thee."

All healing, of course, is of God, regardless what name we may attach to it. Henry Ford's doctor used to say, "We cut them, but God heals them." However, I have chosen the title of this chapter to differentiate between what we know as natural healing from divine healing and miracles. We wish to speak now of healing through nature or natural means.

False Interpretations

I cannot recount the number of times I have read and heard sermons with the above Scripture text used, which was taken completely out of its context. Many well-meaning and godly men have done violence to this passage by extracting it from its setting. We not only make God a liar but we cause poor, helpless people to rest falsely on a promise that God did not make, when we quote a CONDITIONAL promise without the conditions, or by attaching other conditions not in the context (i.e., the Scripture that precedes and follows).

One dear man wrote a tract titled, "Moses' Medicine Chest." He then quoted the closing line of Exodus 15:26, "I am the Lord that healeth thee." He encouraged the readers of the tract to "take God at His Word," and claim Him as Healer. Perhaps the man meant well but he was dead wrong when he failed to quote and take the whole verse into consideration.

With this twisted method of Bible teaching, an atheist can prove that there is no God, for it is plainly stated in Psalm 14:1, "There is no God." But here we must challenge him to quote the context that reads, "THE FOOL HATH SAID in his heart, there is no God."

My dear friend, Dr. R. Fuller Jaudon (now in Glory), for over thirty years pastor of the Tabernacle Baptist Church in Kansas City, Missouri, and who was so well loved and long known as the "dean" of Baptist pastors, recounted this incident: One day he passed a blacksmith shop that had a sign over it which, he said, should be over some pastors' studies. It read, "All sorts of twistings and turnings done here." Let's not be guilty of twisting the Scriptures to the hurt of others as well as ourselves.

The Complete Unfailing Promise

We must challenge those who, as in this instance, twist one sentence out of its context and unconditionally declare, "I am the Lord that healeth thee." Let us read the entire passage, Exodus 15:26.

"If thou wilt diligently HEARKEN to the voice of the LORD THY GOD, and will *do* that which is RIGHT in His sight, and will GIVE EAR TO HIS COMMANDMENTS and KEEP ALL OF HIS STATUTES, I will put none of these diseases upon thee, which I have brought upon the Egyptians: FOR I AM THE LORD THAT HEALETH THEE."

This healing follows NATURALLY, AS WE WALK IN HIS WORD day by day. Although this is a kind of natural healing, yet it is of God. The healing processes go on day and night within our body because we observe His law.

Shortly after my complete 'nervous breakdown,' came the seeming collapse of all the vital organs of my body. In my desperate condition I sought out godly friends and real men of God who believed in divine healing. They were so kind and prayed earnestly for me. However, it did not please the Lord to deliver me in this way. He was shortly to reveal to me this natural plan of healing according to His Word. This process took longer but it taught me patience and endurance. Through it, I have gone from strength to strength and have been given a foundation for sound and robust health that I would never have known otherwise. I cannot thank the Lord enough for revealing this truth that has been a solid rock under my feet for more than forty years. It is this, God's natural healing plan, that I seek to set out in this book and pass on to those of my generation and the ones to follow.

Are you having physical difficulties? This natural healing can be yours, if you are willing to abide by the directives the Great Physician prescribes in His Word as given in Leviticus 11 and Deuteronomy 14. I can bear testimony to these 'keys to health,' having suffered so much and now having tested this divine prescription so many years.

We all have been taught by well-meaning people that these nutritional laws were only for Israel; but there is no premise upon which we can separate the moral and dietary laws of the Almighty. They are both still in force. However, "the proof of the pudding is in the eating." "Taste and see" that all God's laws and ways are good.

Yes, we can claim the promise, "I am the Lord that healeth thee . . . If thou will diligently hearken . . . to give ear to His commandments" [and to His health laws, etc.].

Nature's Danger Alarm System

God has given us an automatic alarm-signal by which natural healing can be regulated. Tonsils are the system's first lines of defense. They act as fuse plugs and as the flashing, red light-danger signals at railroad crossings. When they become inflamed, swollen and sore, they throw up a barricade saying, "Check the foods that have gone down the hatch." By the irritation they are saying, "Don't swallow any more until you do."

Some people have been known to put pennies behind their electric fuse plugs and so making a "blown fuse" impossible. (Incidentally, this is against the law and punishable by fine.) They are ignorant of the fact that this can cause any electric gadget or appliance in the house to be blown out or even the whole house to be set afire.

Is not this what we do when we have tonsils removed? However, we usually treat the symptoms rather than correct the cause.

When parents were about to have tonsillectomies performed on their children, we suggested that they take the children off all pork products including many of the lunch meats, wieners, etc. The condition cleared up, and it took a relatively short time before they were convinced of the wisdom of this action. After several years of "clean" eating, they were never bothered with inflamed tonsils again.

Dr. William Brady in his newspaper column states, "The death rate from tonsillectomy is still frightfully high, frightful to me, that is. For this reason alone I'd never consent to the atrocity in any case.

"Let no one infer that I'm opposed to surgery. I'm quite fond of surgery. If or when I'm the patient and the doctor merely hints—my reaction is, 'Well, what are we waiting for?' Several times I have enjoyed—I mean enjoyed skillful, painless surgery and I'm grateful for it.

"But don't try to tell me tonsillectomy is surgery. No matter who commits the assault, in my opinion it is simply crude, blind dissection of the throat without warrant.

"People keep sending me newspaper reports of fatalities from tonsillectomy, and I wish they wouldn't. I know and you know and the ever-ready operators should know that tonsillectomy is a serious major operation. In too many instances, the victim succumbs to shock, hemorrhage, or 'cardiac arrest' on the operating table or to septic pneumonia or lung abscess from inhaling foreign matter in the course of the operation."

[Whatever technique is used, the *symptom* is treated, not the *cause.*]

Doesn't this sound like true wisdom? Let's not tamper with God's high-precision equipment, our bodies, which the Psalmist David says, "Are fearfully and wonderfully made." Rather let us be careful to follow the instructions in God's manual, the Bible, which will insure its finest, happiest and disease-free performance for many years to come (Exodus 15:26; Proverbs 4:10).

18

Wheat, the Staff of Life

Best Whole Food

"Man shall not live by bread alone but by every word that proceedeth out of the mouth of God" (Matthew 4:4). Here our Lord Jesus Christ, quoting the Word that God gave to Moses in Deuteronomy 8:3, stresses the importance of the spiritual Bread of Life to our heavenly life, as physical bread is essential to our earthly lives. It would follow, since the Creator placed such importance upon bread, that all its original natural nutrients should and must be retained, in order for man to sustain his life healthfully.

Why is bread, made from wheat (with all its original nutrients) called, "the staff of life"? Because our all-wise God and Top Nutritionist placed all the following essential elements in each whole grain: phosphorus, potassium, sulphur, manganese, nitrogen, iodine, oxygen, hydrogen, flourine, lime, magnesium, chlorine, carbon, iron, sodium and silicon. (See page 131.) This is the very backbone of life-substance. Bread in Jesus' day contained all these life-sustaining essentials. They had not made the advances "the wise men" of our day have, in removing this real life-nourishment through refining processes.

There is a substance in the wheat germ called choline, that God placed in the wheat for the purpose of keeping blood

A GRAIN OF WHEAT

A-Honeycomb of Cellulose
B-Starch Grains   C-Particles of Gluten

Phosphorus

Lime

Magnesium

Chlorine

Carbon

Iron

Sodium

Silicon

Potassium

BRAN

Sulphur

Manganese

Nitrogen

ENDOSPERM

Iodine

Oxygen

Hydrogen

GERM Rich In Natural Vitamin Oils

Fluorine

This enlarged cross-section diagram illustrating the structure of a grain of wheat shows that most of the vital body-building elements of the wheat berry are contained in the wheat germ and the bran coatings.

vessels flexible and resilient. Choline in action, serves to burn out the cholesterol, a fatty substance that collects in the walls of the veins, and thus prevents hardening of the arteries with all its attendant evils. Today, however, the heart of the wheat with this substance is taken out, since the wheat germ will spoil if not refrigerated or vacuum packed. Since bread and flour are shipped hundreds of miles and must be kept several days, the bakers could not afford such a loss, so we must take it in malnutrition and impaired health. Other preservatives, such as calcium propionate, are added to prevent further spoilage.

Some preservatives have been found to be dangerous and even cancer producing. We should be wary of anything that hinders the natural physiological processes. How can any chemical, strong enough to keep foods from being 'broken down' though left for months on grocers' shelves, be 'broken down' in the digestive tract and not do some damage?

White Flour Poisoned?

Still worse, however, is the fact that after the heart of the wheat is removed, the rest of the flour is bleached (for white flour) with a poisonous gas called, "Chlorine." May I here refer you to a nutritional scientist, Catharyn Elwood, who, after studies at the University of Maryland and Cornell University Food Science Laboratories, has been acclaimed "America's Leading Nutrition and Health Lecturer." In her book, *Feel Like a Million,* pages 55 and 56, she relates how for twenty-five years, 90 per cent of all the white flour milled in the United States was bleached with "agene," chemically known as nitrogen trichloride.

Sir Edward Mellanby, one of Great Britain's foremost medical scientists, produced "running fits" in dogs in one or two weeks by feeding them a diet containing agene-bleached white flour. The fits became so violent in some dogs that they died.

The Food and Drug Administration of the United States government has now banned the sale of this agene (nitrogen trichloride.) The millers are now using chlorine dioxide for the same purpose. In one of the flour journals we find "chlorine dioxide is more powerful than nitrogen trichloride."

Robbed of Life-Substance

The University of Minnesota tested cattle by giving grain that had been degerminated like our commercial flours. The cattle gained weight and looked wonderful. Then began the inevitable sign of vitamin E starvation. They began dropping over as though they had been shot.

> After evidence like this is shed
> No wonder some wag has said,
> "The whiter the bread,
> The sooner you're dead."

Mr. George Philgreen of Kansas City, Missouri, adds an enlightening bit of testimony out of his own experience. He stated, "Several years ago, I had a breaking out on my body, especially on my hands, face and neck, accompanied by a swelling, with a sticky substance oozing from the sores. My eyes were almost swollen shut. I could not bend my fingers, and my ears stood out from my head like a couple of pork chops. After trying almost every remedy about which I was advised, and going to one of the leading skin specialists in our town and other doctors to no avail, I decided I could use my money to better advantage and went on a fast from food, drinking only water for 24 hours. I would then eat one food at a time. If it did not hurt me, I would continue to eat it. By this process of elimination, I found that my difficulty was due to white sugar and white flour, both of which have been refined. I cut out these two things from my diet and my skin cleared."

Foods such as butter, cream, eggs, and many cheeses are high in cholesterol (animal fat), which is a cause of arteriosclerosis, the depositing of fatty globules on the walls of blood vessels. If this is not checked, high blood pressure will result and ultimately the victim will probably die of some heart ailment. It isn't that the above foods are not good or should be avoided by active people, but the mischief follows because of a deficiency of B vitamins found in wheat, namely choline and inositol which burn up and utilize the cholesterol. When we rob the wheat of this precious element, can we blame the Almighty for the plague of heart attacks in America? Arteriosclerosis is the No. 1 killer today. We have kicked the "staff of life" right out from under ourselves and become the author of our own physical doom. Let's stop trying to improve on the Almighty's food products and start living healthy, normal lives as He intended.

Most health food stores and some regular grocery stores carry 100 per cent whole wheat bread. Be sure it is so marked. This is made from the real whole wheat flour and is usually kept under refrigeration or otherwise not shipped long distances. In cases where preservatives are added, they pretty much nullify the nutritional value of the wheat. Much of the 'whole wheat bread' found in our stores is little better than the white bread.

Home Grain Mills

What can we do to get the nutritional value from the wheat that is so necessary? First, may I suggest: invest in a little home grain mill. A good, sturdy one can be purchased for around $15, depending on the make. If possible, drive out to a farm or to a grain elevator and buy some whole kernel wheat that has not been sprayed with insecticides. It is very inexpensive. It can also be purchased at many health food stores. Then put it (dry) in jars and it will keep indefinitely. Keep a jar of the *whole kernel* wheat in the pantry, to be used (after grinding in the little electric mill) as a substitute for cracker crumbs in meat and nut patties, fish loaves, soups, etc. and sprinkled on various breakfast foods. You can feel the strength of this living wheat through the day, so that you will not feel the need of or have a constant hankering for snacks.

At our house, we fix wheat like 'Cream of Wheat' every morning for breakfast. I heartily recommend this. It will pay off in health dividends. Grind the wheat about 45 seconds. (CAUTION: barely cover the blades—not to over-load = one good serving.) Place in cooking pan—preferably stainless steel, add water and cook about five minutes to desired texture. Salt to taste. (To keep it from being lumpy, mix it with a little cold water first.) It's good with honey or vegetable margarine (the soft type or a little butter if you are 'active'). Parents, there is not a body-building breakfast food in all the world comparable to this. This will 'stick to the ribs' and tell your children from me, it will really "put them in orbit." In the illustration on page 131, you can see all the nutrients and essential elements that whole kernel wheat supplies. This is the Creator's "staff of life."

It is tragic that so many millers have robbed the wheat of its life-substance to the weakening and sickening of men's bodies. Many theologians also have robbed the Bread of God of its divine life to the blinding and destruction of men's lives and souls. In both cases let us keep what God gave in the beginning that we might be well physically and spiritually as John writes, ". . . that thou mayest prosper and be in health even as thy soul prospereth" (III John 2).

A Spiritual Application

Since we live so close to the physical and material, we need to be reminded constantly that God made man A LIVING SOUL. Jesus quoting from Moses declares, "Man shall not live by bread alone but by every word that proceedeth out of the

mouth of God" (Deuteronomy 8:3; Matthew 4:4). God's Word
will do for our souls what food does for our bodies. If we neglect
this, we will be spiritual cripples and we'll wonder, 'What's the
matter with us?'

But what about your spiritual nutrition? Your body is just
the house that you (a soul) live in. As the man (soul) is greater
than the house (body), so the soul-food is more essential than
bodily nutrition. How few even take thought for their spiritual
nourishment, let alone partake sufficiently of the soul-bread
from heaven. Is it any wonder there are so many spiritually
weak, anemic, sick and disabled Christians, who many times
bring more reproach to Christ's Name than praise? Let us also
in this realize the law of cause and effect. If we would be strong
we must partake of the Bread of Life daily.

Hear the testimony of two great men: No man ever suffered
greater loss or went through greater trials and tribulation than
Job. Concerning soul-food he states, "I have esteemed the
words of His mouth more than my necessary food" (Job 23:12).
This is a tremendous testimony realizing that hunger for food
is man's No. 1 craving.

No one ever had a tougher assignment than Jeremiah. (Read
his book.) All his countrymen, including prophets, priests, rul-
ers, and the king turned against him, and had him jailed for his
faithfulness to God. Yet in the midst of it all, he declares, "Thy
words were found and I did eat them, and thy word was unto
me the joy and rejoicing of my heart" (Jeremiah 15:16).

Let us be diligent stewards of both soul and body, and be
careful to fortify both with the bread which our Redeemer-
Maker has provided.

19

White Sugar and Its Danger

Robbed of Choline

Our all-wise and benevolent Creator placed this precious substance we call choline (and inositol) in raw sugar cane, as well as in the wheat germ. Its primary function in the blood is essentially the same as detergent in motor oil. It keeps the blood vessels from becoming clogged by utilizing (burning up as fuel) the fatty globules (chapter 13), insuring normal and smooth operation of the system (taking into account needed exercise and bodily activity—chapter 24).

We, of course, have made strides far beyond the Almighty who formed and fashioned the human body, and who made food for its proper functioning. Our sugar companies take this good natural food product through fourteen steps of 'refining.' In this process we extract the B-complex, the enzymes, proteins, minerals and vitamins. We feed this precious "by-product" of blackstrap molasses to our cattle. We people eat the lifeless remains, white sugar. Result: strong cattle and weak people; healthy animals and devitalized humans.

The insanity of these times is revealed in an announcement that came over the CBS network recently that some farmers have discovered that cattle will eat shredded newspapers soaked in molasses. This means they are not only plaguing the animal with dead pulp, but do they really believe this poisonous ink will not affect both the milk and the meat? Humans have also been fooled with strychnine in orange juice or coffee.

Why did the Chief Nutritionist place choline in the sugar cane? We have found it is needed to utilize the cholesterol, the fatty substance that is deposited on the walls of our veins and capillaries primarily through the eating of animal fats. Through our sugar refining process we are saying, "Lord, you made a big mistake." Most people would not put this in *words* but they do in *actions*. They may not *say* so, but they *live* so. We must get back to the Almighty's natural plan of nutrition if we are to be well, which would include the whole cane sugar and blackstrap molasses. The other alternative is to be ready to pay the cost of sickness, and doctors and medical expense. Today we are taxing the facilities of our over-crowded hospitals and forcing the building of new additions. There is no question that this situation could be much alleviated through proper nutrition and moderation in food consumption.

Starvation Food

Refined sugar is a starvation food for it has been robbed of all its nourishment. It is a starvation food because it satisfies your call for food, but leaves your thousands of cells sick and dying. It will only give you a little quick energy and make you fat. If raw cane sugar is not available, use honey as a sweetener. Dark brown sugar is better than the white.

White sugar is dead. It can be stored in 100 pound sacks for years in filthy warehouses and still be sold for a good profit. Worms will not eat it. It holds nothing for them.

Thief of Calcium

Refined white sugar tends to deplete the calcium in the body. It has never been known for a child or adult who has sufficient calcium and whose blood sugar is not above normal to become a victim of polio. More will be said on this subject in another chapter dealing with colas, soft drinks, etc.

Leading dentists in America are unanimous in their opinion, that the greatest destructive agents in the mouth are the bacteria which live on refined white sugar, which in turn create acids that attack the tooth enamel causing cavities.

Vitamin News reports, "Calcium has so many functions it is hard to say how vital its importance is. There are good reasons to believe that no virus infection can occur unless the calcium levels of the body fluid have dropped below a certain limit. No doubt here is where the insidious relation of soft drinks and ice cream to polio is to be found."

Some health authorities have stated that refined white sugar should be banned from import to our country. Yet the United States is one of the biggest importers of refined sugar. Every 100 pounds of sugar imported displaces 600 pounds of milk or about 500 pounds of potatoes. Even from the standpoint of our own economy this means a loss to our agricultural program. However, it is an ill wind that blows no one some good. Hospitals, doctors and dentists will have a thriving business and, of course, funeral parlors and cemetery associations will come in for their share. This brings the patient and this chapter to an end.

20

Our Devitalized Foods

Taste-Thrill Competition

Food has become such a highly competitive business in America, that each company must find new ways to increase the taste-thrill and appearance through artificial flavorings and colorings. Many try to attract buyers through newspaper, TV and radio appeal, not on the premise of their product retaining the organic and natural vitamins and minerals, but rather on the basis of tickling the taster. The company that can produce the most beautifully packaged and delicious tasting product, especially if he has a big "10 cents off" on the package, will soon have the most popular brand in the whole country. The fact that the product may even be injurious to one's health is of no consequence to most food shoppers. Most buyers mistakenly feel, "Because it is on the market, it must be safe." What about cigarettes?

One day while shopping in a large supermarket, I examined most of the labels on the packaged cookies. I was looking for one that did not have artificial flavorings and coloring. Among all, I suppose a score or more, I found only one, and that was the lowly gingersnap. Yes, even the peanut cookies had artificial flavorings and colorings. The same was true as I looked through the pastries, rolls and bread. Preservatives are also added to retard spoilage. (Check the food labels.)

All America was shocked to read this Associated Press story regarding a widely used food coloring:

Washington, DC (AP)—The Food and Drug Administration is banning Red dye No. 2, once the most widely-used dye in foods, drugs and cosmetics until studies labelled it as a possible cancer-causing agent.

The FDA ban which took effect February, 1976, ended 68 years of use of Red No. 2, although products on sale containing the coloring were not withdrawn from the market.

The last obstacle to the FDA ban was removed when the U.S. Court of Appeals lifted the stay it had imposed just two days earlier at industries' request. New products made with Red No. 2 will be subject to seizure or recall. The dye has been used in hundreds of products including soft drinks, candy, ice cream, cosmetics, etc.

(This is clear evidence that we cannot take for granted that everything on the grocer's shelves or in the butcher's shining white display case is safe for human consumption just because it is there.)

Back in 1960 a report was given to me while travelling through Israel for the first time which stated that no artificial food colorings or flavorings were allowed in that country. They were more concerned about building a strong and well people, than getting an exciting taste-thrill out of every bite of food they ate. This showed in the health of the people as a whole, considering also the fact the government is encouraging the observance of the dietary laws (pages 51 and 52). Now in the later 70's Israel has become more 'Americanized.' Cola's, etc., have been introduced from the States. Israel is being contaminated with American 'strides' of contamination and is learning the ways of the nations.

Embalmed Groceries

Do you remember the old-time peanut butter and how the oil used to come to the top of the jar? It had to be refrigerated or it would become rancid. All live foods must be refrigerated, if they are to be kept any length of time, or they will spoil. We are now so advanced that we have homogenized and added preservatives to most peanut butters, so that it can be kept on the shelf for weeks at a time without 'breaking down.'

Without going into the scientific terms let me tell you what happens. The food is taken through an "embalming" process which does keep it from breaking down. These preservatives are so effective, however, that when the food is taken into the body, even the stomach gastric juices cannot break it down completely as it should. It passes through your system without giving you the needed strength and energy you require. This is also the cause of much undue belching of foods. The "preserved" foods refuse to be broken down by the gastric juices.

Most of our canned foods contain benzoate of soda. This chemical is added to preserve the food. However, in some vegetables, up to 66 per cent of the food value is destroyed. Acid foods such as tomatoes and citrus fruits tend to hold more of their nutrient value than other foods. Benzoate of soda added to canned citrus fruits (pineapple, grapefruit, orange, etc.) has a bad reaction with some people. Some have abnormal amounts of "stomach gas" and on some it will cause a skin rash. While we were in Israel, a Jewish scientist from the States announced he had discovered that certain preservatives used in fruit juices and dried fruit are cancer producing.

The only way to keep your body alive is to eat live foods. EAT AS MUCH OF THE FRESH VEGETABLES, FRUITS, NUTS, GRAINS, etc., as possible. Grains, nuts, and fruits are sun-blest "preferred stock" since they are doubly removed from the soil (which sometimes is defiled by chemical drift in irrigation water, etc.) and doubly protected by nature's own coverings. This was the ideal food before the fall.

The pasteurization of milk destroys about 38 per cent of the B complex vitamins according to Dutcher and Associates. Vitamin C is largely destroyed which means you must get this much needed vitamin in fresh citric fruits, etc. Better take the loss in pasteurization than a chance with diseased raw milk. If you buy raw milk, be sure it is certified (or from a clean farm dairy).

Life-less Foods

Processed cheeses are 'not natural.' They are usually manufactured from one third each of water, gelatin, and cheese, which have very little real nourishment. Be sure any factory wrapped cheese is marked "natural." The regular longhorn, cheddar, Swiss, roquefort, New York sharp, etc., are natural cheeses but should be used wisely, although fat content differs. These often come to the grocer in bulk form, which he cuts and packages in different weights and prices. Cottage cheese is rich in protein and is a wonderful food.

Not long ago, a report in a popular national magazine titled, "A Four Billion Dollar Hoax," revealed another phase and segment of America's devitalized foods. It related how many of our dried breakfast cereals that are dehydrated and devitalized, have very little food value left. Yet thousands of mothers in America send their children away to school or to play, after a bowl of this lifeless stuff, and think they have nourished their children. To be fair, we must give credit to the companies that enrich and fortify their foods to various extents with proper vitamins. More fortunate are the children who have mothers who sweeten such foods with dark brown sugar, or better yet, with raw sugar or honey.

Mothers, if taking these so-called breakfast foods away from your children causes an unconquerable war, may I suggest that you buy wheat germ that is available in all stores and sprinkle this generously on every helping. Again, I urge that you make your own breakfast food from live wheat as suggested in Chapter 18. We need to shout it from the housetop—*"To have live bodies, we must eat live foods."*

If we ate live foods, they would satisfy our hunger, but eating devitalized foods, though we may fill our stomachs, our cells keep crying for the real-life nutrients. The vicious circle continues by eating more devitalized foods until there are big stomachs and lifeless bodies. A tremendous burden is put upon the heart, but yet it doesn't have sufficient nourishment to carry on its work. And so, overeating and inactivity continue to fill our hospitals and populate our cemeteries.

An experienced nurse who worked in a doctor's office a number of years told me, "Seventy-five per cent of the people who come in for medical care are of a class who seemingly cannot afford to eat the proper foods. If they had eaten right (live foods), they would never have needed to see a doctor." It would be wise to cut down on other things first, even clothes or the old family bus. Walking would contribute to better health, and the savings from both walking and unnecessary trips to the doctor, would provide for better and healthful foods. Consider and consent.

Much more could be said about our devitalized foods. One great cause is that our farmers have not obeyed the Scriptural command to let the land rest every seven years, according to the Sabbatic year program. After we have robbed the soil of all its nutrients by continual disregard of this law year after year, we then add artificial chemical fertilizers which allegedly burn up the soil, and which in turn produces more devitalized foods. Poison sprays also take a deadly toll in sickness and early deaths. Therefore, it is possible to have one's stomach full and still suffer from malnutrition. In fact, certain forms of cancer have definitely been found to be caused by malnutrition, a lack of certain essential nutrients. And so, many suffer from *spiritual* malnutrition because they neglect partaking daily of the food from heaven. What about your *spiritual* health? A weak and sickly spiritual state can contribute and even be the cause of various physical difficulties.

"A man's spirit will bear his infirmity but a wounded spirit, who can bear?" (Proverbs 18:14).

21

Preparation and Care of Food

Homemaker's Role

Why do so many homemakers become bored with their daily routine? Why is it so many find their role in life so uninteresting? Without doubt, one reason is because they are not aware of the important position they occupy; first, in bringing forth children and Biblically populating the earth, being co-partner with God Himself in recreating human life. God intended a man's wife to be a true helpmate and a mother. Trouble follows if this plan is disregarded.

What an essential role the wife has as a homemaker. The daily routine of the kitchen can become very monotonous unless one thing is kept in mind; she should never forget that meal by meal, day by day, she is building and molding the bodies of her family. "You are what you eat." She should consider herself an artist, a dietician, a constructor, a sculptor and home physician. She can prepare dishes that are beautiful to behold which help stimulate the appetite. She should study nutrition, and try to serve well-balanced meals so that her family will get all the needed vitamins and minerals, thus putting precious live building blocks into her family's bodies, insuring them against sickness and disease. What a lofty, worthy calling! How tragic that so many are more interested in tickling tasters, than building bodies.

Keep in mind, meal-planner, that these bodies are made up of billions of living cells. In order for your children to grow healthy and strong bodies and for adults to retain their health, they must be fed on that which contains these living (organic) cells. Man is a living organism and he must be fed with that which is (living) organic. The body would soon collapse if fed inorganic substance such as dirt, rocks, sand, etc. Whenever possible include fresh vegetables, fresh fruits, and grains, etc., in your meal planning. Use a minimum of canned foods. If you are cutting down on red meats, supplement your diet with plenty of nuts (almonds, pecans, walnuts, peanuts, etc.), soybeans, sunflower seeds, fish, chicken, eggs, low-fat cheese, etc., to keep up your protein intake. Without such supplements, strict vegetarians are likely to suffer from fatigue and eventually low blood pressure and anemia. A food table guide giving the vitamins, minerals, etc., of the various foods is found in Catharyn Elwood's book, *Feel Like a Million*.

Healthful Cooking

Much food value is destroyed by overcooking and hard frying. It is wrong to cover vegetables with water, boil out the vitamins, pour them down the drain, and eat the pulpy substance.

It is still worse when cooked in porous aluminum which is a relatively soft metal. Even though aluminum were not harmful, still it is unclean. It is impossible to thoroughly clean. The pores become breeding places for germs. Stainless steel cookware, in which the lids fit tightly, makes "waterless" cooking possible. Put just a little water (enough to create steam during cooking time) in the pan with your vegetables and *cook slowly.* This way, you will not destroy the vegetables' vitamins by high temperatures and they will greatly retain their garden freshness.

It is better to undercook than overcook (like leaving the tiny center of the potato raw). By this method, also, you can have two or three vegetables cooking in the same pan without adulterating and intermixing their flavors.

The lower the heat temperature in cooking, the more of the live nutrients remain to feed and build your body. Try it sometime and see the tremendous difference. (If you occasionally burn food, do not throw it away. Your body requires some carbon.)

Do not salt food until after it is cooked (boiled foods) since salt draws out the valuable vegetable juices. Presalting before cooking, therefore, will cause much of these precious juices to be lost.

This word of caution. Wash thoroughly all fresh fruits and vegetables bought in the stores. As a rule these have been sprayed with poisonous insecticides that can be injurious to health. Besides, they have been handled by many people, perhaps some carrying "unfriendly" germs and even contagious diseases. At our house we wash them with soap and water. I would suggest you do this before you place them in your refrigerator. Soap is one of the best antiseptics, but rinse thoroughly. During deadly cholera epidemics, caused by contaminated foods, the people are warned to wash all vegetables carefully and to avoid unclean and questionable foods.

Balanced Meals

Homemaker, since you are fashioning and molding the bodies of your family, take the time to study the various elements these bodies need. They are primarily made up, first of all, of PROTEIN found in nuts, grains, soybeans, meats, fish, chicken, eggs, milk, low-fat cheese, etc. PROTEIN means "that which comes first." Then, the body requires greens—rich in

VITAMIN A. All sorts of vegetables, especially carrots and apricots are good sources. There must be VITAMIN C, found in citric fruits: grapefruit, oranges, lemons, limes, etc. "C" stands for cement, that holds the body together. Don't forget CALCIUM from milk, cottage cheese, etc., that builds good strong bone structure and teeth, and will also fortify you in old age from fractures as results of falls, etc. VITAMIN B_1 and B_2 of course are necessary, that come from wheat, soybeans, yeast, etc. VITAMIN E appears to be a real wonder-worker, i.e., from the natural organic source— wheat germ oil.

Remember, lard is a killer. Use all-vegetable margarine such as soy, safflower, and corn oil, since this will aid in burning out the cholesterol, the fatty globules, that have collected in the walls of your veins. I would suggest the soft type which is less hydrogenated. Best foods may cost a few cents more but you may deduct it from your pill bill.

Unfortunately most margarines have preservatives which not only fail to contribute to one's health but can be detrimental. If you have doubts as to the quality of the brand you are using, it might be wise to use small amounts of butter, rather than clog your body, which is God's temple, with undigestable foreign matter.

Helpful Hints

Keep your food from oxidizing. If you leave lettuce 'out in the air,' it begins to wilt. The oxygen in the air actually begins to burn it up and destroy the living tissue. It will soon be worthless as food. This is true of most all living foods. This is why pure natural corn oil becomes rancid if not tightly capped and refrigerated. (If bought in large quantities, pour into smaller air-tight bottles.) Keep butter refrigerated in its foil wrapper. Vegetables should be kept tightly wrapped in plastic or foil. Real live whole wheat flour should be refrigerated as any live food.

See that your family gets some fresh fruit every day. It (plus ample walking) is the best laxative for natural bowel action. For in-between snacks for the children, keep some 'peanuts and raisins' on the table. In fact, mixing them together makes a delicious treat. Popcorn is a 'not bad' food: season with hot corn oil and salt. Especially if a person is overweight, salt should be kept to a minimum. However, in hot weather more salt is necessary to replace salt lost in perspiration. It creates thirst and retains liquids in the body. (See page 117.) Nuts of all sorts are good. Keep ice cream at a minimum. It is mostly sugar and actually acts to deplete the system of its calcium.

This tip to those who may be weight conscious. God has His own "built-in" weight adjuster in nature. Since the human body is made up primarily of water, it has much to do with a person's weight. Generally, fruits that have multiple seeds have a tendency to hold liquids in the body whereas single-seed fruits cause the body to give them up. (Most extra-ripe fruits act as a laxative.) If overweight, do not give up multiple-seed fruits completely, for the Vitamin C in citrus fruits is an essential. But make the balance largely single-seed fruits; among these are the peach, apricot, plums of many kinds, prunes, etc.

No. 1: When sugar is added to these fruits and juices, it nullifies the weight-reducing properties. A mal-active thyroid gland can also be a contributing factor in weight control problems.

If underweight, then major in the many-seeded fruits such as apples, grapes, oranges, etc. This does not mean you can disregard other common-sense means of keeping your weight balance, but it is definitely a help.

No. 2: Adult health will improve and weight can be reduced by cutting out between-meal snacks. Give your heart a rest-break and live longer.

The best exercise for weight reducing should be taken about three-fourths through every meal. First, put your hands on the edge of the table in front of you, push back firmly, stand up and walk. . . . away, especially away from every rich dessert, pies, pastries, ice cream, etc.

The Lord created saliva in the mouth and gastric juices in the stomach to break down food, so that it might be assimilated into the various parts of the body. Drinking with meals dilutes the stomach acids so they cannot digest the food properly. Gas is formed, then pain and finally, "get the bicarbonate." This is why it is so essential that you make a rule at your house—"Do not wash the food down." Chew it well. Suggest that if any are thirsty that they drink at least thirty minutes before the meal; and it is best to wait 1½ to 2 hours after meals. Washing meals down with drinks is the cause of much stomach discomfort after meals, and can lead to serious physical disorders and illness.

If stomach ailments persist after observing all common-sense health measures, cut down or leave off condiments. After all, isn't it an insult to the flavors God has put in the various foods to drench them with all sorts of dressings and sauces, etc.? These usually contain artificial flavorings, colorings, and pre-servatives.

Darkhorse Chocolate

We have put chocolate on our "dark-brown list." Though not habit-forming in our candies, cakes and drinks, yet it does contain stimulants. Experiments have proven that cocoa and chocolate actually prevent calcium from being assimilated in the body. In other words, by taking chocolate with milk, it actually destroys the value of the latter. To build bone and teeth, eliminate or use chocolate sparingly. There is a good substitute found in health food stores called "carob" that is healthful. It comes in candy bars and other forms that children will enjoy.

A friend of mine who served as a missionary in Africa said that natives there would eat the bean of these cacao trees. He stated that if for some reason they were unable to secure this bean, they would "be as doped and worthless." Chocolate contains 2.2 theobromine and some caffeine.

*NOTE: The cacao is a sterculiaceous tree. Sterculius was a pagan god that presided over manuring, dung—in allusion to the foul odor. The dried and partly fermented seeds (cacao beans) of this tree are chiefly used in making cocoa and chocolate. They yield a yellowish fat used in candy, etc. (Webster's Dictionary).

Chocolate does give you a lift temporarily and seems to warm the very cockles of your heart and imparts that sort of "cozy feeling." But may I reiterate that any stimulant that lifts you above your normal emotional level will afterward drop you below it and actually leave you feeling lower than before you imbibed the pick-up. Let's feed the nerves instead of 'whipping the tired horse.'

We would here make a suggestion to candy manufacturers, in the light of growing public awareness of proper nutrition, that chocolate-substitute, "carob," candy be made available in bars and packaged for the general market. It is available in most health food stores.

Perhaps by now you have said to yourself, "I'd rather be dead than give up all these things." But, would you rather be sick and half dead? Each one of us has the prerogative to decide this for himself. I must admit that being the possessor of good health does not come along the fast and loose line of least resistance. Discipline is the trademark of life's most valued possessions.

22

From Soft Drinks
to Soft Bodies

Polio Prevention

The president and founder of Polio Prevention, Inc., states that he has often told his son that he would rather see him take a drink of whisky than a bottle of the cola drinks. This sounds strange coming from a father who never drinks hard liquor. Why such advice then? Because, he says, the boy knows whisky is wrong, from the first taste unto the final destructive results. Not so with the colas. The hidden lurking evil in them is masked with its heavy load of delimed white sugar. Do children (or most adults) realize that this subtle delectable drink is made up of phosphoric acid, sugar, caffeine, dye and flavoring matter and slowly but surely is eating away and destroying the very foundation of their health? Phosphoric acid is made by treating phosphate rock with sulfuric acid; can it be that people drink such a mixture? Phosphoric acid—px pH 1.8, commonly contains impurities such as silica, iron and aluminum, arsenic (an accumulative poison) lead, fluorine, etc.

Phosphoric acid breaks down the body lecithin, causes brain fag, neurasthenia, nerve breakdown, physical apathy, mental irregularities, anemia, polycythemia, acidosis, renal (kidney) lesions, rickets, faulty calcification, a marked shift in bone structure, unsuccessful reproduction, tetany and prevents the normal increase in size of growing children.

Such a drink as this opens the door to polio. This strange insidious chemical combination decalcifies the entire body. If the body has sufficient calcium and if the blood sugar is not above normal, polio is well nigh impossible.

Polio blood is low in calcium and invariably low in iron—possibly due to phosphoric acid preventing absorption of iron by forming insoluble iron phosphates.

The Council of Foods and Nutrition of the American Medical Association stated, "The Council believes that carbonated beverage should not be sold on school premises. There is merit also to the suggestion that attempts be made through school boards to place a zone around school buildings, in which the sale of candy and soft drinks would be prohibited."

Dr. V. P. Sandler, U.S. Government physician and author of "Diet Prevents Polio," stated, "I firmly recommend that the sale of all soft drinks be prohibited in schools, both elementary and high schools. I firmly believe that this prohibition will be an effective measure in the prevention of polio."

Since 'an ounce of prevention is worth more than a pound of cure,' it would follow that it is wiser to build strong, healthy bodies fortified against disease than to inoculate weak, sickly bodies with various vaccines.

For Good Teeth

The American Dental Association also condemns the sale of candy and soft drinks in schools.

The Rhode Island Dental Society recommends the ban of soft drinks in all schools.

The journal of the Connecticut State Dental Association published a very informative article showing pictures of children's teeth that had been ruined by the habitual use of colas. The

Association called upon the state school officials to remove and bar the cola-vending machines from all public school buildings.

Paul Harvey, radio news commentator, reported on Tuesday, February 10, 1976, that dentists in West Germany have stated that candy should be barred from public schools and a warning put on the wrapper that it is harmful to the health.

You ask, "What *can* we drink?" Wonderful, refreshing, cleansing, healthful water, with such an enduring taste that really satisfies the thirst.

If there is any question about the healthfulness of your drinking water because of pollution or by overchemicalization, don't take a chance. Spring water and distilled water can be purchased relatively cheaply in most grocery stores. In times of natural disaster when normal sources of water are defiled, remember to boil it before drinking.

Discipline yourself to drinking water between meals instead of thinking you must have a drink of 'pop.' Why pour a load of sugar into your blood stream each time you are thirsty, thickening the blood which can trigger off any numbers of evils? Of course there are times for other drinks such as one of God's own mixtures of body-building food drink—milk. Think of the many fruit juices—orange, lemon, lime, grape, grapefruit, apple, apricot, prune, etc. *Get them fresh* if possible. Citric canned juices are not best for you.

We appeal to the beverage industries to follow the example of those in the State of Israel, to make available bottled noncarbonated fresh, fruit juice drinks. Because of the increase in health education, there is a large growing potential beverage refreshment market that is, as yet, untapped.

Coffee?

Of course I am constantly asked, "What about coffee?" Yes, I know how delicious it can be—I am a Swede. However, it is common knowledge that there is no food value in caffeine. It is habit-forming. Remember, a stimulant that lifts you above your normal emotional level will afterward drop you below it, thereby making it a depressant. Coffee will give you a real "pick-up" and a feeling of exhilaration temporarily. Some of the little irritating problems seem to drop away. However, after it has run its course in two or three hours, it will drop you below that norm and "let you down." In other words you are "whipping a tired horse." And after the ride the horse will be still more tired. Don't forget, you are the horse. If you must have coffee, keep it at a minimum. Boiling brings out the tannic acid, so drip or silex rather than percolate. In the event of the slightest heart disorder, cut out coffee immediately. If you want a hot drink in cold weather, try hot caffeine-free drinks.

The Harvard University never deals with trumpery. It is the oldest (founded in 1636) and was the first, privately controlled, full-fledged university established in the U.S.A. and has remained at the top ever since. No department or professor there can be charged with being alarmists.

However, the Harvard University School of Public Health and the Department of Epidemiology has issued a warning about the possibility of coffee causing cancer in the *lower urinary tract*. They do state that one third of this type of cancer is likely to be attributable to coffee drinking. The least that can be said regarding tests of *bladder cancer* is, "The conclusion reached is only that the relationship between coffee drinking and bladder cancer warrants investigation."

Another reminder: Take your drinks between meals. If you insist on drinks with your meals, sip them slowly so as not to dilute your saliva and stomach gastric juices to the slowing down of your digestive processes and eventually to the injuring of your health.

Cigarettes

Cigarettes are still worse, not only in their harmful effects and offense to others, but because of their convenience to always have them on one's person. As soon as the depressive action sets in from the former stimulation, another can be taken until the smoker becomes inveterate. He is caught in the vicious circle. As a friend of mine told me, it was very easy for him to give them up, "I've quit over 50 times already."

Even before the Surgeon General's report, a famous doctor stated, if there were one-tenth the evidence that the Brooklyn Bridge was unsafe for travel as there is that cigarette smoking causes lung cancer, it would be closed within one hour's time.

Britain's Royal College of Physicians, which never deals with trivia or sensationalism, made a study on smoking and health. The report revealed this evidence: "Cigarette smoking is a cause of lung cancer and bronchitis, and . . . contributes to . . . coronary heart disease. . . ."

The report goes on to state that "Cigarette smokers have the greatest risk of dying from these diseases and the risk is greater for the heavy smokers." Why be a sucker?

From our own country, consider this report by Edward Edelson which appeared in the New York *Daily News:*

CATASTROPHE COMING, SAY CANCER SPECIALISTS

NEW YORK—"And now for the next problem," said Bruce N. Ames. "The coming catastrophe."

Standing in his small corner office at the University of California in Berkeley, Ames is talking about cancer, so matter-of-factly that the meaning of his words doesn't sink in immediately.

"The United States is really heading for a disaster," he said. "I'm convinced of it. They may pass a Toxic Substances Act, and get people to stop smoking, but most of it is too late. I can name you more than 20 possible catastrophes, chemicals that are in widespread use and may be carcinogenic [cancer-producing]. Just one or two have to be real, and we're in for real trouble. . . .

"For one thing, cancer specialists see just such a catastrophe unfolding right now. It is the catastrophe of cigarette smoking. Cigarettes are blamed for 80% of the 93,000 cases of lung cancer that will occur this year. Cigarettes are associated with an increased incidence of cancer in the mouth, throat, pancreas and bladder. More than 100,000 cancer deaths annually—nearly 1 in 3 of all such deaths in this country—are associated with cigarette smoking."

If Ames is right, his test will give, for $200 and in a few days, better information than standard animal carcinogenesis tests that cost $100,000 and run for more than three years.

At this point, so much documented evidence has been revealed and confirmed in a report by the Surgeon General of the United States and from other authoritative sources that cigarette smoking causes cancer of the lungs as well as many other ailments including 'heart trouble' . . . that any further proof is superfluous.

23

The Scientific Mosaic Laws

The Rev. Thomas H. Nelson, former president of the American Bible School, editor of *The Ram's Horn,* and author of *The Gospel of Cause and Effect,* in his book titled, *The Mosaic Law in the Light of Modern Science,* states, "After submitting the Mosaic law to the most rigid tests of modern scientific standards, the writer is convinced that Moses himself is a true modern—a radical scientist of the most advanced school. He is even seen to be leading most of our present day scientists in the popular and important studies of bacteriology, psychology, physiology, hygiene, botanic chemistry, practical eugenics, sanitary sciences, quarantine principles, zoology, geology, astronomy, etc." We are aware, of course, that Moses was divinely inspired.

The philosophies of great men such as Socrates, Plato and Aristotle are now out-dated. Who now follows the exact therapeutical advice of Hypocrates, yet the laws of Moses are as up-to-date as when they were written over 3,500 years ago. His system of laws and sciences has been made the very foundation and chief bulwark of the most advanced modern nations. There is no portion of the commandments of God in general or of the Mosaic code in particular, that is not based on a scientific understanding of fundamental law.

The most modern research proves that not one command of

the original law can be rejected without the offenders suffering physically or mentally. In this Gentile dispensation of grace (Ephesians 3:1,2), only spiritually speaking is it true that "Christ is the end of the law . . . for righteousness . . ." and that "We are not under law but under grace." There is only one matter in which the law of God is null and void, and that is in obtaining salvation, righteousness and eternal life. There is only one city and land to which we can travel without law, and that is heaven. In every other sphere, on every other level, and in all other cities and lands the laws of God are in force and are as sure as the law of gravity.

Let us consider some of these laws that are ignorantly passed off many times as mere "ceremonialism." Let us not be guilty of casting away God's unchanging laws, which the Apostle Paul states are holy, spiritual, just and good.

Running Water Hygienic Bathing

Let us examine some of these laws in the light of modern science. The law commanded that every Hebrew must wash his clothes and bathe his body in running water after handling diseased or dead people or other polluted things (Leviticus 15:13). Why, particularly, in running water? Now, after thirty-five hundred years, science has discovered that much disease is contagious and some infectious and is transmitted by infinitesimal bacteria, millions of which may attach themselves to the hands and bodies of those coming in contact with them.

These disease bacilli live in etheral media and are hatched out and multiplied by the body heat of the one receiving them, and thus diseases both contagious and infectious are spread. To wash in a bowl of water, after the first dip, is to wash in polluted fluid full of deadly germs, leaving many of them still on the hands and the body when the bathing is finished. But when the bathing is done in running water, they are constantly being carried away so when the bath is finished, the hands or body are free from the diseased bacteria.

Bodily Contagion and Infection

If a Hebrew sat on a seat or saddle where a leper or a man with an issue or running sore had sat, he was pronounced unclean and required to wash his body and change and wash his clothes and go into isolation outside the camp from one to seven days.

The seat or saddle that was so contaminated must also be cleansed by water or by fire and then thoroughly aired. Why? Especially because the light and gauzy clothing of that warm country admitted the body of the uncontaminated person into immediate contact with the diseased serum and germ, and then the bacteria began to feed upon the victim's body, hatching out new batches by the very heat of his body and so contagions spread, and if on an open sore, by infection. This was made impossible where the Mosaic law on purification was kept and honored.

Sanitation

If a Hebrew worked in the field, he was to carry a paddle with which he was to dig down and cover any waste or offensive matter that was left by him. As late as the Spanish-American War, we have an illustration of the result of disregarding this Mosaic law of hygiene. Because this sanitary regulation was not observed, the lives of many of our American soldiers were lost. This is another corroboration of the soundness of the scientific Mosaic laws. In some heathen countries, where this particular law is disregarded, the air becomes so poisoned with infectious bacteria that the poor natives die off at times with plagues and pestilence, like flies in a winter frost. No, this law has not become obsolete. It is still in force.

The Sabbath Rest

Time and space forbid our even touching on the many other various laws given for our very survival, blessing and happiness. The moral, as well as the dietary law which was given for man's welfare (not his salvation), could also be proven to be scientific.

For instance the infidels of France, after the revolution, changed the Sabbath, or rest day, from the seventh to the tenth day. However, their horses and mules could not stand this unnatural arrangement. They soon became diseased and died so rapidly that scientists were appointed by the government to investigate the cause. They found that a return to the seventh day principle was necessary to physical welfare, health and long life. These animals broke down because they were taken out of the harmony of God's law that was written into the very fiber and fabric of their being. And so, as someone has said, "The donkeys taught the atheists a lesson in practical theology."

Talmage reminds us that "Our bodies are a six day clock and if they are not wound up on the seventh, they will run down to the grave." The following experience happened to a dentist friend of mine. He said God revealed to him a new way of reading X-rays through which he could detect infection seeping into the lymphatic channels from a diseased tooth, though it showed no local pus pocket. By extracting certain teeth and draining gums, great cures were being effected.

One day he told me it was necessary for him to be in his office seven days a week. I said, "Doctor, this is not good: you are working contrary to the law of God which was given for man's welfare; violators pay a costly price."

He explained, "Yes, but I am doing good and helping these people."

"I understand that," I replied, "but God has written this law of one day of rest out of every seven, into the fiber and fabric of our being. It is engraved in the very organs of our bodies. As batteries need constant recharging, so our bodies need regular periods of rest. These laws cannot be broken; we only break ourselves over them."

It was only a matter of time before my doctor friend began taking drugs in order to keep going. Then greater tensions and weariness called for more narcotics. In a comparatively few years, he had a complete mental and physical breakdown and had to be taken to a mental hospital where shortly afterward he died.

The command, "Six days shalt thou labor," is just as important and binding as the need for one day of rest. It has been proven that health and true happiness are impossible in idleness. The adage, "The idle mind is the devil's workshop," is not just an empty saying. Idleness breeds idiocy and work makes for wisdom.

Think of the men among your own acquaintances who have died shortly after they retired. The exception lies with those who have become active in some other field, interests or hobbies. Men who refuse to accept a life of idleness, generally keep right on going strong into ripe old age.

Cecil B. DeMille stated, "Many of us will be forced to retire at some future time but it is an insidious word. It means, according to the dictionary, 'to withdraw from action, from circulation; to designate no longer qualified for service.' " He himself was a man of tremendous action. Addressing law enforcement officers one time he stated, "Man has made 32,-600,000 laws but hasn't succeeded in improving on the Ten Commandments." Those that observe the law of, 'Six days labor and one day rest,' will reap the benefit of it: those that don't, pay the consequences.

Circumcision

God ordained circumcision as a token of the everlasting covenant between Himself and His people Israel (Genesis 17:9–14). It is scientifically significant that the babies were to be circumcised on the eighth day after birth. The following quotation from recognized medical and nursing tests, confirms the wisdom of our Heavenly Father and Great Physician, in setting this particular day in the life of the newborn infant for the day that circumcision was to take place:

"The prothrombin (substance in the blood necessary for coagulation) level decreases in all infants during the first few days of life, and blood clotting time is prolonged. Hypoprothrombinemia (lack of substance in blood necessary for coagulation) is most marked between the second and fifth postnatal day... Spontaneous recovery usually occurs in seven to ten days" (Van Blarcom, Carolyn Conant, Obstetrical Nursing, 4th edition, New York, McMillan Co., 1957).

God's command to circumcise on the eighth day is still more proof that all His laws are scientific.

Law of Tithing

There are other laws mentioned in the Bible, such as the law of tithing. This law did not originate on Mount Sinai. The Patriarch Abraham paid tithes over four hundred years before the law (Genesis 14:17–24). After Abraham refused the spoils of Sodom but paid tithes to Melchizedek, God said to him, "I AM thy shield, thy reward shall be exceeding great" (Hebrew—Genesis 15:1). Jacob also observed this law of finance as recorded in Genesis 28. He went down to Lebanon a poor man and came back twenty years later wealthy. The law was incorporated into the Mosaic economy as given in Leviticus 27:-30–34. Malachi further expounds the blessings and curses that follow those who observe or disregard this statute. The contention that tithing was only given to Israel, as some contend about the dietary law, is being constantly disproved by those who put tithing to the test. Others unwittingly suffer reverses for failing to observe it.

Cyclone Mack, the old southern evangelist, used to say, "It's as impossible for you to tithe and not prosper, as it is for you to stand out in the rain and not get wet."

We offer this law as another evidence of the fact that all of God's laws are still in force. They were never made to give us heavenly eternal life, but to bless and prolong our earthly mortal lives. Let us thank God for them.

Millions of God-fearing people through the centuries, and multiplied thousands in this generation, could testify to the blessing of observing the law of tithing. Like the moral and dietary law, it was never repealed; it is still in force and we can, and many do, enjoy the prosperity and blessing of it today. Our going to heaven doesn't depend on our observing this or any other law (Romans 3:28). What an uncertain and flimsy hope that would be. Our salvation lies in Christ's righteousness, not our own. We 'broke' the law and came under its total condemnation. Christ kept the law completely and bequeathed to us His transgressionless righteousness. He died in our place on earth that we might share His place in Heaven. Now, through simple *faith* in Christ, I inherit all He is in God. I now possess His legal standing in heaven before God. Paul declares regarding our salvation, "Therefore it is of *faith* . . . to the end the promise might be sure" (Romans 4:16). Have we digressed in our thinking? No, all things gravitate to the Redeemer. He is the center of the universe. "He is before all things and by him all things consist" (Colossians 1:17). "All things were made by him and without him was not anything made that was made" (John 1:3).

Let us be eternally thankful that salvation lies not in our works of the law but in Christ's work on the cross. Still, may we heed our Creator-Saviour God who cries out with compassion, "Oh, that there was such a heart in them, that they would fear me, and keep *all my commandments* always THAT IT MIGHT BE WELL WITH THEM and with their children forever" (Deuteronomy 5:29).

The Dreaded "Fall-Out"

The greatest and most foundational of all the health laws the Lord God Eternal ever gave us is the one found in Leviticus 17:11, "The life of the flesh is in the blood." Not only is 'the life of the *flesh* in the blood,' but also the life of all members of our bodies—the eyes, the brain, the lungs, the entire 'man.'

Parents, if you want your children to have a good growth of hair on their heads, do not cut off the blood supply by tight fitting caps and hats. An airforce officer told how he lost his hair by wearing a tight-fitting helmet. The pressure compressed the blood vessels between the skin and the skull, cutting off the hair's 'life-line.' Periodic massage of the scalp, to keep it loose and free for the tiny capillaries to do their work, is also essential for healthy hair and to avoid the dreaded "fall-out."

24

Profitable Exercise

"Bodily exercise profiteth little [yet it profiteth], but godliness is profitable unto all things, having promise of the life that now is, and of that which is to come" (I Timothy 4:8).

In Line of Duty

"Godliness is profitable unto ALL THINGS," and the "all things" necessarily includes bodily exercise. When we speak of exercise, we usually think of bodily activities outside our regular routine. Today we speak of walking as exercise, but not so with the Apostle Paul or the early disciples. Walking many miles a day was to them just a part of their daily life and duties of "godliness," in carrying out the great commission. It is recorded in Acts 20:13 that Paul chose to walk from Troas to Assos (about fifteen miles) while the other disciples went by boat, "minding himself to go afoot."

Since living in the land of Israel and knowing something of the terrain of the country, we know they got plenty of "bodily exercise" walking and climbing the hills and mountains of that very rugged country. Even riding a donkey or a mule gives one a good workout.

Considering all this, Paul contends that this sort of exercise has only "promise of the life that now is." Since they obeyed the laws of God and enjoyed the natural and organic foods that had not been devitalized as ours, plus getting plenty of exercise, sunshine and fresh air in the line of duty, they did not have the problem of malnutrition and attendant physical ills that we know today. They could rightly advise, "Don't major in the minors" since at that time the 'minors' were part of their regular duties. In this book, I only seek to call us back to "nature-al" nutrition and health measures that the Lord God planned for His creatures in the beginning.

Danger of Insufficient Exercise

One of the great sins today is gluttony. As we have related, many dig their graves with their teeth and commit suicide with the fork, knife and spoon. The average American consumes great quantities of rich foods of all kinds. Instead of burning up this energy by walking and other bodily activity, he sits and watches TV for hours and drives the car to the grocery store if it's only half a block away, using power steering, power brakes, etc., to keep from using the muscles God gave him. He must have a power mower he can ride to keep from panting and puffing from over-eating. Men used to golf for the exercise to strengthen their muscles and tone up their bodies; but now Mr. American plays the game on a motor scooter so he can be fashionable and have a heart attack. Therefore, power steering, power brakes, power windows, power garage doors, etc., etc., are *musts,* for he *must* guard against over-exertion because of a weakened heart due to a lack of proper exercise and exertion.

What is the result of all this soft living? Soft muscles in general and flabby heart muscles in particular are the greatest danger of all that lead to the marble orchard, the city of the dead. It is a universal law: "What we do not use, we lose." This is true of our body's muscles. When body resistance against disease germs goes down, before too long, food starts coming up; weakness, colds and sickness come on. When food is not burned up by bodily activity, it lies in the stomach and intestines and decays and soon manifests itself in various discomforts: dyspepsia, gas pains, and later in ulcers, abnormal growths such as tumors, etc. Do you think it strange that you feel tired as though you had been 'gassed' when you awake in the morning, after putting such a heavy load on your heart by eating hamburgers, peanuts, popcorn, etc., just before retiring? You thought you were resting but your heart put in a full day's work. Breakfast means to "break the fast" which should have begun after the evening meal. Even a bedtime snack for the children should never consist of any more than a glass of milk, a graham cracker, and the like. For the best health, adults, no between-meal snacks.

Clogging the System

During America's celebration of our bicentennial anniversary in 1976, Benjamin Franklin was frequently quoted. We need often to be reminded of his classic statement, 'Keeping clean within and without is the secret of health.' I believe it can be safely said that most all who are in the hospitals for treatment or for surgery (barring victims of accidents, infectious poisoning or contagious diseases) are there because they have clogged their minds with negative thoughts or clogged their physical systems by eating too much or bad junk foods. If we ate right and less, we would not have to work so hard at exercising in order to keep weight down, would live life on a much higher, more carefree and happier plane and so get much more accomplished.

Babe Ruth, the home-run king, died in what should have been his prime years. Why? Ask Ty Cobb. He writes in his autobiography, "He [Babe] starts shoveling down victuals in the morning and never stops. I've seen him at midnight, propped up in bed, order six huge club sandwiches and put them away, along with a platter of pig's knuckles and a pitcher of beer. And all the time, he'd be smoking big, black cigars.

"Next day, he'd hit two or three homers and trot around the bases, complaining all the way of gas pains and a belly-ache."

What might he have done if he would have taken even normal care of his body?

"Activate or Disintegrate"

You are fortunate if you have a job that calls for physical activity, use of arms and walking during the day. You may not feel the need of further exercise. If you are an office worker, use every opportunity that you have to get up from your desk. Instead of scooting your chair and passing those papers, get up and walk. If you can do favors for others that call for bodily activity, do it.

Why did Mr. Jones die of a heart attack shoveling snow? Because of flabby muscles (skeletal, abdominal and diaphragmatic) due to lack of exercise the rest of the year. Putting a sudden load on the weakened heart muscles is more than it can stand. To make matters worse, Mr. Jones started shoveling snow right after a heavy meal. The heart had already had an extra load put on it by pumping an extra blood supply into the stomach to help digest the food. Now a double load is put on the heart by taxing it beyond its capacity with violent exercise. Moral: no strenuous exercise immediately after mealtime and regular moderate exercise the rest of the year.

Vigorous exercise now and again is beneficial if you are in good general health. A fast walk, jogging, pumping uphill on a bicycle, playing tennis, etc., forces the blood to the farthest extremities of your body, into the tiny capillaries carrying its life-giving load to and restoring and replacing the decadent cells. This accounts for the flushed cheeks, etc., after some energetic physical activity. This also enforces deep breathing that increases the intake of oxygen, so stepping up the body's efficiency.

CAUTION: Remember, no strenuous exercise immediately after meals.

Parenthetically, take some vigorous exercise immediately after a hot bath, especially in cold weather, to guard against the common cold. End the bath with as cool water as possible: this will "close the pores." The exercise will get the blood circulating well throughout your body.

Dr. Paul Dudley White, President Eisenhower's heart doctor, who did a grand job in bringing him out of his weakened heart condition after his coronary attack in 1955, recommended bicycle riding as a means of strengthening and toning up the entire system. Dr. White said, "I would emphasize soundness of body, mind and spirit—all three. Too long have we allowed ourselves to be dominated by psychosomatic or 'mind over matter' philosophy, with little concern for somatopsychic or 'body over spirit' physiology. Yet, there is no doubt that good physical health affects the spirit as much as a good spirit affects health."

It is essential that we keep the body in good tone by proper exercise. The condition of the body affects the mind and spirit, and the attitude of the mind and spirit affects the body.

It is no wonder that many children and adults suffer from fatigue and loss of appetite when America's favorite sport is sitting in front of TVs for hours at a time. The Almighty meant for arms and legs to be used in profitable activity. If you don't use them you will lose them. The Creator was speaking of a basic, physical principle when He said to Adam, "In the sweat of thy face shalt thou eat bread [food]." Sweat is related to strenuous exercise, without it your food-eating days will be fewer. Never forget it. . . . "Activate or disintegrate."

Precious Eyesight

It has now become common knowledge that our TVs are glorified X-RAY TUBES. Dangerous radiation has been found to be at such a 'high level' in certain colored sets that they have had to be recalled, and warnings have been given by authorities over the large networks regarding the physical harm that could result from viewing these 'turned on sets that could turn you off.' This means that TV could not only warp minds and souls, but also damage brain and nerve tissue as well as actually destroy molecular body cell life. The purpose of X-RAY treatments is to kill enemy cells. If great care isn't taken, friendly cells can be destroyed which has happened and in some cases are fatal. Can there be, then, some connection between children being such ardent 'TV fans' and so many having to wear glasses today? A young man friend who was a 'heavy viewer,' began having spells of blindness. He took our gentle warning and the difficulty cleared up. An older friend, a constant 'watcher,' noticed a very rapid increase in blindness. If we belong to the Lord, let us remember we are not our own, only stewards of this house, the body. We have an obligation to take care of it. May a word to the wise be sufficient. See that your children get plenty of exercise in the sunlight, not left to disintegrate under the rays of the TV. (With all the TV improvements it is still not wise to sit too closely and directly in front of the set.)

It is also very possible that when Paul wrote, "Godliness is profitable unto all things," (I Timothy 4:8), he could have been referring to the Spirit of God actually quickening his body making it vibrant and even vibrate. We read that Moses on Mt.

Sinai trembled and quaked as he experienced the mighty power and presence of the Almighty. Many believers through the centuries have had similar experiences as they have realized God's mighty presence. One religious group in the past century spoke of this as "the shakes," which, when the unbelievers witnessed, they trembled with fear. It was this experience that gave the Quakers their name.

Peter Cartwright (born in Virginia, 1785) was in the vanguard of the pioneer Methodist preachers in America. Many in his meetings had the experience known as "the jerks" and to such a degree that "fine bonnets, caps and combs would fly," a work attributed to a genuine manifestation of God's Spirit. (Cartwright did say some excitable people counterfeited it.) The Ultraorthodox Hassidim of the Jewish faith express their desire to worship God even with their bones by bending forward and back rhythmically as they worship the Lord. All this can truly be said to be 'godliness that profiteth even to exercise.'

"Bodily exercise profiteth . . . and has promise for the life that now is," and being well in body helps us to serve the Lord more acceptably and joyfully.

25

Why Fast?

Questions Considered

"What about fasting?" is a question that is frequently asked.
"Where is it taught in the Scriptures?"
"When and why should we fast?"
"Is it for Christians today?"
"Does this mean taking no food and no water?"
"Could it be injurious to your health?"
"What are the benefits of fasting?"
"How long should you fast?"

Since this book is not a special treatise on fasting, we will touch only a few of the highlights. The spirit of fasting is revealed in Isaiah 58:6–12. It is not to be made a subject of display (Matthew 6:16–18) and should be as unto God (Zechariah 7:5). Fasting should be accompanied by confession of sin and followed by a new obedience to God and His Word, and a renewed yieldedness and abandonment to His Spirit (II Chronicles 7:14; Isaiah 55; Zechariah 4:6).

Biblical Examples

Examples of fasting are many in the Scriptures, such as:
In the Old Testament
David—II Samuel 12:16 and Psalm 109:24

175

Nehemiah—Nehemiah 1:4
Esther—Esther 4:16
Daniel—Daniel 9:3
In the New Testament
The disciples of John—Matthew 9:14,15
Anna—Luke 2:37
Cornelius—Acts 10:30
The early Christians—Acts 13:2
The Apostle Paul—II Corinthians 11:27

Jesus

Jesus fasted prior to each time that He was to make a big decision. He told His disciples that there were certain things that could only be accomplished by prayer and fasting (Matthew 17:14–21). The disciples of John chided Jesus because His disciples did not fast. He said as long as the bridegroom was with them, they need not fast. But the time would come when the bridegroom, Jesus, would depart and then His disciples would fast. This certainly refers to us and this age.

Early Church and Methodists

One secret of the power of the early Methodists was their fasting and praying. John Wesley, in a sermon on fasting in 1789 said, "While we were at Oxford, the rule of every Methodist was to fast every Wednesday and Friday in imitation of the primitive church.

"This practice of the early church was universally allowed. 'Who does not know,' says Epiphanius, an ancient church writer, 'that the fast of the fourth and sixth days of the week —Wednesday and Friday—are observed by Christians throughout the world?' "

Not Easy

Since food is the "No. 1" desire of all the earth, it follows that fasting is not easy. We must also remember that Satan hates fasting. It was evident in his first attack against Jesus in the temptation in the wilderness (Matthew 4:1-4). After Jesus had fasted 40 days, Satan queried, "If thou be the Son of God, command these stones be made bread." Jesus then quoted Deuteronomy 8:3. Satan attempts to break down a person's will in this regard, to keep one from the spiritual victory and blessing that will follow. We must have a firm resolve and ask God for strength to overcome these attacks. Satan can also imitate symptoms and magnify any little obstacle that may arise. He would exaggerate hunger pangs, weakness and even sick feelings, whispering that fasting is not for you.

Expression of Love and Faith

We must also keep in mind that we have a battle with the flesh itself. It is easy for Christians to rationalize when it comes to the appetite. Since hunger for food is the greatest of all man's desire, it dominates all life on the face of the earth. Is it any wonder, then, that many would like to eliminate fasting from this dispensation and say, "It is not for us today"?

A complete fast, of course, is to go without food and water. If you feel you cannot go without the latter, then drink that which is absolutely necessary. Fasting clears the mind and makes it easier for you to think and to pray effectively. Solomon wrote, "All the labor of man is for his mouth" (Ecclesiastes 6:7). When you fast you are saying to God, that He, and the desire to know and do His will, means more to you than the greatest desire of man on the earth.

If the British government was cognizant of Gandhi's fasts, and was moved to action by them, how much more our loving faithful Lord is aware of, and is also moved to answer, the fasting and praying of His redeemed children.

I can add my testimony that I have never truly fasted and waited upon God without receiving a very definite answer and blessing.

Physical Benefits

We need also to consider the physical aspects and benefits of fasting. Needless to say, any truth that is inspired by the Spirit, and anything recommended by our Lord, could not be injurious to our health but will rather be a blessing. Regular periods of fasting help to burn up the superfluous tissues lodged in our bodies—in the intestines, stomach, etc.—that have not been used up through normal activity and exercise. It gives the heart and other vital organs, that are constantly carrying on their work of digestion and assimilation of foods, a much needed rest. It is like turning off the motor of your car and coasting down-hill.

Some people experience a sort of weak, sick feeling when they fast. With no food in the stomach to draw on, the system begins to call on and burn up these superfluous tissues, fats, sugars and poisons which, when pulled into the blood stream, sometimes set up a very unfavorable reaction. Sipping a drink of water and a brisk walk in the fresh air or other physical activity will, as a rule, dilute these wastes and aid the bodily processes so that this sickish feeling is overcome. This is evidence you have plenty of energy stored up. It needs only to be called into action. On a prolonged fast slow down your activity the third day. Fresh air also helps.

We 'advanced moderns' have a problem that the 'less-enlightened' believers of former ages knew nothing about when they fasted. They could fast three days and three nights without food or water without any difficulty. Today in the second day of fasting, our bodies begin to call on and burn up and pour into our blood streams poisons in our food that come from synthetic fertilizers, insecticides, food additives and preservatives, artificial coloring and flavoring, so foods can sit "unspoiled" on the grocery shelf for many weeks before they are bought and eaten by unsuspecting customers.

Therefore, it is almost essential in a fast today to drink water beginning the second day to flush out all these poisons that give the 'fastor' a sickish feeling as this process of elimination is going on. Also if you have not been a 'water drinker' and therefore have but little reserve of the choice liquid, the blood will tend to thicken during a fast, which will slow you down and make you feel weak to the point where drinking water is a must. This feeling is not a sign of lack of food. After getting these toxic wastes out of your system, you will feel much invigorated and even years younger.

I would recommend fasting to all Christians, and especially urge all fulltime Christian workers to imitate the early Christians, by fasting on Wednesday and Friday until 3:00 in the afternoon. (There may be special times when it may be expedient to suspend this rule temporarily.) Then, there should be special times of fasting for an entire day, perhaps two even three days as the Lord may lead. A fast of two or more days should not be broken with heavy foods or a large meal, but rather with fruit juice or perhaps a slice of bread and a glass of milk. The longer the fast, the more carefully and gradually it should be broken.

Above all—"And whatsoever ye do in word or deed, do all in the Name of the Lord Jesus, giving thanks to God and the Father by him" (Colossians 3:17).

Increase of Food Enjoyment

Incidentally, homemaker, if the matter of preparing something different for the dinner table becomes a problem at times, and the members of your household feel that the meals have too much "sameness," you will be surprised how fasting will be a real practical help, just as a "side product." In fasting, as your mind becomes clearer to pray, it also is easier to think even of down-to-earth matters such as home duties. Though some members of your family may take a dim view of fasting two meals twice a week, even skipping one meal will sharpen their appetites and give them a greater appreciation for the food our Lord so abundantly provides. Fasting will also bring out the various wonderful food tastes that we fail to appreciate because of over-eating (which most all people are guilty of). Let us remember that the Almighty is as practical in His works of physical creation as He is righteous in His acts of spiritual redemption. As in tithing there is a financial blessing promised, so in fasting there is a physical blessing experienced.

Fasting's Painless Surgery

When Rev. Edward B. Christiansen of Omaha, Nebraska, joined our staff in Wichita, Kansas, he was suffering from a severe and painful growth on the lower part of his spine. A surgeon informed him it must be removed and a date was set for an operation. He was told no assurance could be given him that he would be permanently relieved or cured, and also that it would be necessary to make monthly trips to the doctor for about three years. . . . (at a pretty penny!).

I would not ordinarily encourage anyone to disregard the advice of a competent, dedicated doctor or surgeon. However, in this case, I did suggest postponing the operation since no definite and lasting help could be promised and because I firmly believed Ed could be healed of this ailment by observing the Scriptural dietary law, and with proper exercise and common sense health measures. Among these was the mild fastings Wednesday and Friday till 3:00 P.M., giving opportunity for poisons and superfluous tissues to be burned up. Fasting is God's key to natural painless surgery. We then rebuild normal healthy cells by proper eating.

After careful thought, since it was not a matter of 'life and death,' Ed decided to postpone the operation. (We do not offer this as a general directive for every spinal difficulty, however.) That was back in April 1963 and now, over 13 years later, it is still 'postponed' because through 'God's key' the door to health was opened and the ailment disappeared and has never reoccurred. In April 1966 Ed married Coral Van Koevering and they now have a fine son and daughter.

Note: I would also recommend Dr. Herbert M. Shelton's book, *Fasting Can Save Your Life* (inexpensive paperback— available at many 'health food stores.')

26

Sunshine

"For the Lord is a sun . . . no good thing will He withhold from them that walk uprightly" (Psalm 84:11).

Our Miracle Sun

All life on earth would soon wither and die without the light and heat of the sun. Sunshine is essential to the absorption of the life-giving nutrients. Make your own experiment. Plant some carrot seed outside in the (full day's) sunshine. Then plant some inside in a box in a dark corner of the basement. Water both of them regularly and watch the results. What is true in plant life also holds true in human life. If a plant cannot survive without sunlight, can we suppose as humans that we can remain well and strong without it?

We will not attempt to tell of all the blessings that emanate from the sun. Its power defies description. As the center of our solar system, it holds all of the planets whirling in orbit at terrifically high speeds. Talk about speed! The earth travels at 67,000 miles per hour or once every 365 days around the sun, and we are held in its grasp as though an eleven-inch steel cable were attached to every foot of the earth's surface. Our minds cannot comprehend such power.

Under dateline of January 1976 the following press article

appeared in the *Wichita Beacon and Eagle,* Wichita, Kansas, USA:

"Washington (UPI)—The first [U.S. official] extensive testing of solar energy to heat and cool homes will begin this spring, Housing Secretary Carla Hills said.

"Solar energy originates from the sun and would last as long as life itself, compared with diminishing fuels such as oil and coal which are pumped or mined from the earth.

"Solar energy would also reduce U.S. dependence on high-priced imported oil, which contributed to the recession in 1974-75 by spurring inflation and cutting consumer buying power.

"Mrs. Hill said experiments will be made in 143 homes, apartments and condominiums in 27 states."

Private contractors are already building solar-heated and cooled homes in Arizona and other states. This will be a great boon healthwise, eliminating burning up of oxygen through fires, as well as eradicating poisonous monoxide fumes.

Type of God

Scientists tell us that earth-launched man-made satellites, powered by energy received from the sun alone, can be kept hurtling indefinitely through space in orbit around the earth. The sun, which is a symbol and just a tiny reflection of God's power, is the source of all physical life and light and every earthly blessing. The Scriptures set forth the sun as a type of the Creator. "The Lord God is a sun. . . ." The sun is the very physical expression of the principle and person of God Himself (Psalm 84:11). As God is the Giver of all life, so the sun is the instrument He uses to sustain all earthly life.

Physical Benefits

Nutritional scientists have called one element of blessing in sunshine, "Vitamin D." It is absolutely essential to the absorption of calcium into the system, and calcium is essential to building of bones and teeth, as well as being a nerve builder and tonic. To insure against broken bones in old age, see that you get plenty of calcium and sunshine to absorb it. Remember, sunshine produces energy. Without this Vitamin D, your body does not burn its sugars.

Often I have seen people waiting for a bus, on a normal sunshiny day, holding a newspaper or an umbrella over their heads, or standing under a canopy to avoid the rays of the sun. They wouldn't think of treating their plants this way. Most of us do not have much time for sunbathing, but let us get as much sunshine as possible. (Exceptions—not at mid-day in summer or too long exposure.) Especially if you are sickly, invest some time daily in the sun. It pays good dividends. (Unhappily, some have a physical condition that prevents much exposure to 'ole sol.')

Vitamin D is found in a few foods, but its supply should not be dependent upon these foods only. Some is found in egg yolk and in milk, and more in the summer than in the winter. Sunflower seeds are wonderful. Reports of improved eyesight, calmed nerves and diminishing (even vanishing) arthritic pains have been reported through the regular use of sunflower seeds. Grind them up in your mill and use all sorts of ways instead of cracker crumbs, in patties, meat and nut loaves, soups, etc. They, mixed with raisins, make an excellent snack for children.

Authorities tell us there are healing rays in the sun to heal every disease. This is intimated in Malachi 4:2, "The sun of righteousness shall arise with healing in His wings . . . unto you that fear my name." It is common knowledge that sunshine (plus fresh air) is the best medicine for colds and tuberculosis. Some report cataracts removed from bathing in the sunshine; first just five minutes with the eyelids closed, then increasing the time from day to day. Eyes were made for the sunlight, not to be hid behind dark glasses. (Exception: on all long drives facing the sun.) In olden times, when prisoners were placed in a dungeon without light for a matter of years, they lost their eyesight —their eyes withered away. Your eyes were made for the sunlight (not artificial light). Work by it as much as possible.

Sunbathing Caution

If you are not used to sunbathing, let wisdom guide you by beginning with just 15 or 20 minutes at the most for the first time, and then increase the time each day. Do not start as a "beginner" in the noon's summer sun; use wisdom. You may prefer to be working in the yard at the time, but keep in mind the importance of turning one side and then the other toward the sun. Do not take a soap and water bath just before bathing in the sun. Let the natural oils of the skin protect you. If the sun is unusually hot, apply a vegetable oil, preferably olive oil (not artificial sun-tan dyes). After sunbathing, give at least three or four hours for the absorption of this Vitamin D into your body, before bathing with soap and water.

Spiritual Application

Above all, remember the sun is only a small type of Him who is the true SUN of Righteousness, the Redeemer-Messiah. After Moses received the law we read that his face so shone when he came down from Mount Sinai, from being in the presence of the Eternal, that he had to put a veil over his face (Exodus 34:29–35). So let us take time each morning to spiritually bathe in the presence of God by reading His Word and spending time in prayer, that others may "see and take knowledge that we have been with . . . the Sun of Righteousness." We, ourselves, will be strengthened and fortified for the journey and we cannot help but bless others with the radiance of His inborn presence. Amen.

27

The Breath of Life

"The Lord God . . . breathed into his nostrils the breath of life and man became a living soul" (Genesis 2:7). A dead body, plus "breath," equals a living human being.

Life's Substance

You may live two weeks without water, and you may live three weeks without food, but you cannot live three minutes without fresh air. God gave you lungs for one reason, and that is to take the oxygen out of the air and put it into your physical system. Every vital process in the body is dependent on oxygen for its efficient performance. The more oxygen you have, the more pep, the brighter your color, the keener your mind and the smoother all your body's functions will be.

Breath is the stuff of which life is made. It is inter-related to the very soul of man, the real life-principle. God formed man of the dust; his whole body was there in its entirety, but not until God "breathed into him the breath of life" did man become "a living soul." Therefore, we know the spirit enters the body at birth, simultaneously with the breath.

The Apostle Paul in speaking of our spiritual new birth writes, "God hath sent forth the Spirit of His Son into your hearts crying, 'Abba [that is], Father' " (Galatians 4:6). When does the spirit leave the body? At death. At Jesus' death we read, "He cried with a loud voice and said, 'Father, into thy hands I commend my spirit,' and having said thus, He gave up the ghost" (the breath of life). As Stephen was dying, he said, "Lord Jesus, receive my spirit" (the spirit of life).

Our life's breath then, is a perfect type of, and inseparably attached to, the very spirit of life itself. God has vested it in an element called oxygen, and bounded it by a physical law.

A Physical Necessity

When a man drowns, his oxygen supply is cut off and his life is ended in a very few minutes. Shut yourself in an airtight room; the same thing happens, and you will be dead in a relatively short time. During the winter months many people are asphyxiated because of unventilated gas stoves. Sometimes entire families have lost their lives in this way. Others prefer to commit unintentional suicide on the installment plan, by asphyxiating a few cells at a time through poor or scarcely any ventilation in their homes. They do it on the premise of being thrifty, of saving money by using less heating fuel. Believe me, it is poor economy.

See that your house is well ventilated. An ordinary furnace in a moderate size, three bedroom house, will burn the equivalent of three rooms of oxygen an hour. It will be a good investment in your own health to see that this amount of fresh air is supplied. By failing to do this, you are robbing your own body cells of the real life substance, and to that degree suffocating them and greatly lowering your own resistance to sickness and disease. What you think you save in fuel will soon be going out in doctors' and medical bills, and maybe funeral expense. So many learn the hard way.

One winter, a number of years ago, I was conducting an

evangelistic campaign at Bronough, Missouri. I was given a room on the third floor of a residence in which I was to stay during the two weeks of meetings. There was no outside ventilation whatsoever. I was unable to open any of the windows and there was no outside door. The only heat was an unventilated gas stove. Not many days passed before my body was actually suffering from suffocation. The result—I took one of the worst deep-seated colds I had had in many a day. Believe me, it was no help to the campaign.

This is not an isolated instance. It will happen every time that you are robbed of the precious substance of oxygen. Later, I experienced the same thing in similar situations, and I saw the pattern of another physical law. Of course, there are other ways to lower your resistance and take colds and other diseases, but the above is one sure-fire method. I also found that I could head off a cold, if it were caught in time, by taking a long, brisk walk in the fresh air, taking special thought to inhale deeply.

Very Important

A humidifier is an absolute must to protect against winter 'colds.' We make "hot-house plants" of ourselves by drying out the tiny alveoli (air sacks) in our lungs (that extract oxygen from the air and put it in the blood stream and that give off carbon dioxide) with the inside warm, dry air in our houses and buildings, and then plunge them into cold, damp air by going outside. The results are sickishly obvious.

America's New Killer

Emphysema (due to lack of oxygen) continues to take an increasingly greater toll each year. Air-tight homes and cars, now both in winter and summer, contribute victims. Some think all heaters and coolers bring in fresh air. This is not so.

On a real cold or hot day it would be impossible to effect the inside temperature without reheating or recooling the same stale air. Remember, cold air is not necessarily fresh. So we leave our oxygen-starved houses to get in our oxygen-less "stale air-conditioned" cars. But the end is not yet with the pollution of city air by motorcars below, and jet planes above, belching poisonous deadly monoxide gas. The monoxide of one VW midget auto was the first killer of hundreds of Jews by Nazis in Germany. Now we commit suicide on the installment plan.

You must have an ample supply of life-giving oxygen to keep well and alive. If you have a choice, live where there is plenty of vegetation and as far off the busy street as possible. You cannot wake up feeling 'like a million' in the mornings unless you have oxygen (fresh air) galore during the night.

Suggested Note

(If you live on a busy, heavily trafficked thoroughfare, keep your front windows closed especially during times of heaviest traffic and get fresh-air ventilation by opening windows in the rear of the house or building. Remember also, because the air is cold does not mean that it is fresh.)

A 1976 news report from the Associated Press, New York, states:

"Dr. Walter Blumer of Netstal, Switzerland, said he had 75 patients who died of cancer over a 12-year period, and 72 of them had lived within 50 yards of a state highway carrying 5,000 vehicles a day through Netstal.

"He said this meant the death rate from cancer was nine times higher among those living close to the highway than among those living beyond."

God has provided for the refurnishing of oxygen in the action of photosynthesis that takes place in plants, as they burn up carbon dioxide (exhaled from our lungs) and give off oxygen. The more plants you have in your home the better. Here again, let us follow the way of the Lord and wisdom for our good and His praise. (Read "How to Be Fit at Every Age," from Aerobics —*Reader's Digest,* March, 1968.)

"Green thumb" secret: Do not over-water plants, or you will suffocate and rot the roots. Put gravel or sand in bottom of plastic pots for 'breathing.' Water from below if possible or from one side. Plants' roots need oxygen.

(It is distressing to see more and more beautiful trees, vegetation, flowers and grassy meadows destroyed to make way for more cement and pavement in man's onward march to conquest and success.)

Beauty, Voice and Poise

Beauty specialists tell us that increased circulation brought about by good breathing will do more for the complexion than a lifetime of massage. Psychoanalysts say that an inferiority complex may result from something as simple as a lack of proper breathing and fresh air. Good radio announcers realize the importance of proper breathing to voice quality and control. Experienced public speakers know the value of deep breathing and its importance to platform poise and voice power.

Red Cheeks, Robust Health

Properly inflated lungs right the body as ballasts right the ship. Remember, your lungs go down to the waistline, but unfortunately most people use only the upper part of their lungs. They are like a motor struggling along only on half of its potential power. Is it any wonder they feel half dead?—They are. Make your own test. Take a quick breath, filling your lungs clear down to the waistline. If you get an "oxygen-jag," a light-headed feeling, it is proof that you have not been breathing properly. Whenever you can and every time you think of it, take a deep breath of fresh air way down to the waistline. Soon you will do this more and more until it becomes "second nature." If you take up biking you will automatically breathe deeply pumping uphill, or in doing any other rather vigorous exercise. This is good, for it forces the blood into all the tiny capillaries and the body's extremities, flushing the entire system, putting you on the road to robust health.

Breath-Holding Easy Heart Test

Dr. H. L. Herschensohn, M.D., states, "Among the many procedures used by a doctor to determine the condition of your heart is the breath-holding test.

"Take a deep breath [of fresh air] and hold it as long as possible. Time it with your watch. A stop-watch would be better. As a rule, a healthy person can hold his breath at least twenty seconds. Some can hold it up to a minute or even longer.

"If, however, you find you cannot hold your breath fifteen seconds, then it would be advisable to see your doctor for whatever other tests he thinks necessary to determine the condition of your heart."

As I mentioned previously, some have written asking if the author is still alive and inquiring about the condition of his health. The answer to the first question is, yes. To the second question, if the above test is any criterion, I have just held my breath for a solid 60 seconds, which I believe is a good recommendation for faithfully following the truths of this book as I have the past 40 years. [I would advise against holding the breath too long, i.e., beyond the point of normal endurance.] Now in 1976 I feel like a 'kid,' work at a stand-up desk all day long, never have headaches, pains and aches, etc., that plague many who contend that these truths are foolishness.

Your Car Breathes

When driving in the mountains and in high altitudes, why is it that your car doesn't have the power it ought? You have plenty of gas and spark, but it doesn't have the get-up-and-go. The reason, we say, the air is thinner. The higher the altitude, the less pressure per square inch, so the carburetor doesn't get enough fresh air (oxygen) with its gasoline mixture to create proper combustion. So if driving any length of time in the mountains, an adjustment can be made on the carburetor. Now, if plenty of fresh air is a "must" for the proper and efficient operation of a gasoline motor (as well as to the growth of plants) how much more essential it is to the healthful functioning of our bodies.

Did you ever stop to think that every part of your body's "motor" must also have a constant supply of fresh air (oxygen)? In Chapter 21 (Preparation and Care of Food) we mentioned that food will oxidize if left out in the air—it wilts. The oxygen actually begins to burn it up. This is necessary in the bodily processes as the blood picks up the oxygen from the lungs and carries it to the stomach, where it aids in the breakdown and assimilation of the foods, so that there is proper "combustion" and smoother operation of your physical vehicle. So, don't be surprised at being half dead if you are not getting sufficient fresh air (oxygen) which converts the food to energy. If your blood doesn't have sufficient oxygen (plus proper exercise) the food lies in the stomach and decays, leaving you sluggish and sick.

An automobile must fire on all cylinders if it is to operate smoothly. If one or two spark plugs are disconnected, it can be noticed in its poor performance, especially under a strain. If you are chugging along like an automobile firing on half its cylinders, then it's time to check up on yourself. Remember, for every effect there is a cause. All of life, including our bodies, operates according to set laws. If any one of these laws are disregarded, we will have difficulty. Fresh air with the precious element of oxygen inhaled into the lungs is another of these "spark plug" laws, that must be observed for the smooth operation and health of the body. Resolve today that you will no longer cheat your body, the temple of God, of the precious, yet free and untaxed fresh air He has so lavishly given. Every moment that you live, partake to the full of the "breath of life."

Miscellaneous Notes:

WARNING: Lack of fresh air (oxygen), i.e., insufficient amounts in the human lungs for an extended period, *can cause permanent brain damage.* This can result in mental deficiency and subnormal brain control. (With the advent of air-conditioned cars we are subject to the danger of breathing even more deadly fumes since the motor is kept running even when the car is not in motion, to keep our 'hot-house-plant' society comfy.)

28

Restoring Sleep

"He giveth His beloved sleep" (Psalm 127:2).
"The sleep of a laboring man is sweet" (Ecclesiastes 5:12).

Rest for the Heart

Sleep acts as a generator that charges the battery of our bodies. It is as important as good food, exercise, fresh air and right thinking. It is like putting your car in neutral, idling the motor and coasting down a hill and getting momentum for the next one. Wouldn't it be foolish to put your car in neutral going down a hill and at the same time to speed up your motor, burning gasoline uselessly and putting extra strain and unnecessary wear on your motor? This is what some people do by eating before retiring. Instead of letting the heart rest, (idling the motor) during the night, they put a tremendously heavy load upon it by forcing it to pump extra supplies of blood to the stomach to digest the new load of food. Is it any wonder they wake up the next morning feeling as tired as when they went to bed? Their poor heart has been overworked all night long. Some have less consideration for their hearts than cruel slaveholders did for their slaves. Slaves were allowed to rest during the night. How do you treat your heart?

Key to "Good Morning"

The Creator, according to the Scriptures, divided life's time segments into day and night; the days into hours and the night into "watches." The day was reckoned from sunrise (6:00 AM by timepiece) to sunset (6:00 PM) as the third, sixth and ninth hours. The third hour, three hours from sunrise, 9:00 AM; the sixth—noon; and the ninth would be 3:00 PM. Generally there were three meals during the day at intervals of about five hours beginning with breakfast. The nights were divided into four watches. The first from 6:00 PM to 9:00 PM. The second from 9:00 to midnight, etc. Watchmen were set over the cities at this hour to stand guard against possible invaders, fires, etc., while the people slept. This was a period of twelve hours when no meals were served. So the first meal in the morning was called "breakfast" which broken apart means—"break fast." This fast period gives the body opportunity to burn up its waste tissue and to rest. As we have cautioned, if any food is taken before retiring, it should be very light. Milk is a wonderful nerve tonic and food (but a 'weight-gainer' taken at bedtime). Save your wake-up fruit juices for the morning. To wake up your freshest best, by-pass that midnight snack.

Good Bed a Must

A good firm bed is essential to a restful night of sleep. A good mattress is one of the best investments you can make in this area for the health of your body. Better go in shabby clothes than sleep on a poor sway-back mattress. The latter puts a strain on joints, ligaments and muscles and causes impingement of the vertebrae and nerves of the backbone. The result—waking up with a backache and feeling completely fagged out which could trigger other difficulties.

With most people, sleeping on the left side puts extra pressure on the heart. You can check yourself by listening for the pulse-beat with your ear on the pillow. It's better to sleep on your back or on your right side.

Sleep in Dark Hours

Authorities tell us that two hours of sleep before midnight is equivalent to four hours afterward. Therefore the four hours of sleep from 10 PM until 2 AM is equivalent to that of the six hours from midnight until 6 AM. Why? As night comes on and we revolve away from the sun, there seems to be almost a mystic pull down to mother earth that induces sleep and restores man's mental and physical powers. Also there is the stark reality of an exceedingly high 'noise level' during daylight hours in this modern age of zooming jet airliners, trucks, buses, autos (with loud mufflers), motorcycles, power mowers, blaring radios, TVs, which takes its toll on sleep and sleeper. We are also reminded by our Lord that we "are children of the day; we are not of the night nor of darkness" (I Thessalonians 5:5). It is for our blessing to take this spiritually and physically. We are aware in this complex day that many must work at night, and we wish their day-sleeping to be the exception to the rule. The adage, "Early to bed and early to rise makes a man healthy, wealthy and wise," is more than just a pithy saying. Most "greats" have been early risers.

Biological Clock

During our several years' stay in Israel, one way we kept in touch with world events and news from the States was by listening to the *Voice of America* during our dinner hour. One interesting weekly program that followed the news was titled, "Science in the News." One of these broadcasts of particular interest was called "The Biological Clock."

Dr. Carl Hamner of the University of California made a study of the influence of the earth's turning on its axis once every twenty-four hours and its dominance upon all living things including plants, birds, animals and humans. He discovered as darkness came on there was a strange pulling-down force that affected all life. We can only briefly relate how this affects the human body.

Dr. Hamner discovered that during the daylight hours human cells divide more and faster, the bodily temperature is higher; the glands are more active and make more chemicals during the daylight than at night. Some men in the Arctic made a volunteer test by staying in a warm dark room where it was impossible to tell day from night. They first began working in daylight hours and slept at night. They then began working and sleeping at all hours, some working more at night than in the day. But regardless of the time they worked or slept, the body parts themselves did not change—they all functioned as though they knew the difference between day and night. In other words, the men's bodily parts knew what time it was though their minds did not know day from night. Dr. Hamner stated this was a secret that "nature" has not revealed though man has made such great strides in the various fields of science here in the later 1970's. This is more evidence of the marvelous and unsearchable wisdom of God in creation. This is also strong reason why we should work during the day and sleep at night. Take note, "night-owls."

We ought to take a lesson from the birds and chickens. Our Maker created us to function at peak efficiency during the daylight hours and with greater ease. The Almighty designed the eyes to operate in daylight, not artificial light. Let's not try to improve on the plan. His ways are perfect.

Parents, keep in mind that growing children need more sleep than adults. If you, as an adult, feel you need more than seven or eight hours of sleep, check on your diet and elimination. If you feel a nap is necessary during the day, take it after the noon meal, but do not "over-sleep." Too much sleep can make you as groggy and unresponsive as insufficient sleep. In fact, your wits will be sharper and your mind keener by a little under-sleeping rather than over-sleeping. Solomon warns, "Yet a little sleep, a little slumber, a little folding of the hands to sleep: So shall thy poverty come as one that travelleth, and thy want as an armed man" (Proverbs 6:10,11). "Love not sleep, lest thou come to poverty; open thine eyes, and thou shalt be satisfied with bread [food]" (Proverbs 20:13).

But to enjoy the blessing of sleep to the fullest, do a good day's work as unto the Lord, the Greatest, for "the sleep of a laboring man is sweet."

The Best Nightcap

And finally, "Let not the sun go down upon your wrath" (Ephesians 4:26). Balance the ledger at the close of each day. You may sleep, but it will not be the restful restoring sleep that you need if you harbor an unforgiving spirit, resentment, jealousy, envy, etc., in your mind and heart. A troubled conscience has not only robbed many of healthful sleep, but it can be a factor and contribute to all sorts of ailments and troubles of the nerves, mind and body. Getting things right with God and man (husband, wife, friends, neighbors) has been the means of many healings. Keep in mind, our eternal salvation depends on Christ's work on the cross, but our joy and usefulness depend on our walk and obedience to His Word and Laws.

"He giveth His beloved sleep," when we are trusting Him as our "watchman," not the locks on the doors or the dog and the lightbulb in the yard. "Except the Lord build the house, they labor in vain that build it: except the Lord keep the city, the watchman waketh but in vain" (Psalm 127:1,2). Negative thoughts cannot live long in the mind of the obedient, faithful, God-fearing Bible reader for "Great peace have they that love thy law and nothing shall [trouble, stumble] offend them" (Psalm 119:165). Commit it to memory.

29

Sleeping Pills
and Tranquilizers

Tragic Results

In 1950 when tranquilizers came out, the American public was told that they were harmless and safe. Since that time, a different story has been written—in the emotional, mental and physical wreckage of many of its victims. Airplane crashes have been traced to pilots taking tranquilizers (according to a *Reader's Digest* article, July 1962). In hundreds of clinical cases, existing emotional illnesses were aggravated by tranquilizers. In many scores of cases, the victims of tranquilizers developed tremors as is characteristic of the Parkinson's disease. Those who go on taking tranquilizers finally become irresponsive and are not fully conscious of the realities of life. As Dr. Frank Orland warned in the *American Medical Association Journal*, "He no longer has any worries, no longer plans logically, tends to make impulsive decisions, may manifest defective reasoning and, as a result, may find himself in real difficulties." Think of this. Late in 1960, a professor at Columbia University's College of Physicians and Surgeons estimated that, "One in every seven Americans is taking tranquilizers as an escape from anxiety." What must the number be now in the latter 70's?

Deforming Thalidomide

Back in 1961 a tranquilizer containing thalidomide, which was popularly sold throughout Europe, England, Canada, and Australia, resulted in the malformation birth of thousands of babies being born without arms, legs, and even some without either arms or legs. It was also disclosed that over 1200 physicians in America bought the drug to use in experimentation (using people as guinea pigs). Word had just been received of the death of a mother in New York who had taken this tranquilizer during pregnancy. Moments before dying, she gave birth to a baby whose both arms and legs were deformed. What a price to pay for tampering with God's natural laws.

Did some of these mothers take the drug to sidestep the Scriptures, "I will greatly multiply thy sorrow and thy conception"? Most took the pills to be rid of morning sickness and such discomforts. But "The Scriptures cannot be broken." We, in disregarding them, break ourselves over them.

What does all this mean? Nest feathering, perhaps, at the cost of physical breakdown, permanent disability and premature death. Food and drugs are the biggest businesses in America and the most competitive. Why should any industry take chances by gambling with the health and very lives of the people through incomplete experimentation? Doesn't this bear out again the Scriptural warning, "The love of money is a root of all evil"?

Necessary Precaution

What can we do in these matters? Remember the adage, "An ounce of prevention is worth more than a pound of cure." Having a knowledge of these things, let us act accordingly so that it need not be said of us, "My people are destroyed for lack of knowledge," or that we "have rejected knowledge" to our hurt or destruction.

There are many who think because a product is on the market, it is therefore safe and has the blessing of the Food and Drug Administration. Experience has proven this to be a false premise. The blighting and deforming tranquilizer, thalidomide, was sold on the open market without prescription in Europe. It was only by a chance reading that Dr. Frances Kelsey kept it from a large scale market here in the U.S.A. Because of the terrible thalidomide tragedy of thousands of armless and legless babies born, other drugs are now coming under questioning as to their side (and full) effects.

Many also seem to think that all medical doctors are infallible. Experience also proves this assumption to be untrue, although we may wish all of them to be fine, totally dependable and dedicated men. Let us believe that most of them are. However, thousands of the thalidomide tranquilizers and sleeping pills were ordered at the hand of a doctor's prescription.

The Christian's Tranquilizer

Gospel ministers, also, should be completely trustworthy but unfortunately there are some who are not, and some are charlatans. Just so, there are some great and wonderful physicians and surgeons who should be trusted completely, but there are some who are not so well qualified, and some are quacks. The good, the mediocre and the bad will be among us as long as the world stands. Let us pray for wisdom to discern.

By and large, the God-fearing believer's tranquilizer is the Word and Spirit of God. *"Great peace* have they which love thy law: and nothing shall offend them [shall be an obstacle]" (Psalm 119:165). "Thou wilt keep him in *perfect peace,* whose mind is stayed on thee: because he trusteth in thee. Trust ye in the Lord for ever: for in the Lord Jehovah is everlasting strength" (Isaiah 26:3,4). "I will not leave you comfortless," said Jesus. "And I will pray the Father and He shall give you another Comforter [the Holy Spirit] that He may abide with you forever" (John 14:16–18).

"Now the God of hope fill you with all *joy and peace in believing,* that ye may abound in hope, through the power of the Holy Ghost" (Romans 15:13).

"In nothing be anxious; but in every thing by prayer and supplication with thanksgiving let your requests be made known unto God. And the *peace of God,* which passeth all understanding, shall keep your hearts and minds through Christ Jesus" (Philippians 4:6,7).

Special Note: Isn't it unwise to dull a sorrow with drugs in a crisis such as when losing a loved one in death while family and friends are there to help? When the drug wears off and these human hearts and helping hands are gone, the 'victim' is left to bear the sorrow alone which leaves him in even a lower emotional state.

We owe much to the Pure Food and Drug Administration as a watchdog guarding the public against many harmful products. However, it is a human organization and the best of watchdogs sometimes fail. High Christian conviction counts the body God's temple and such things as cancer-producing cigarettes, hard liquors, and other products, etc., are harmful and yet they are accepted and sold on the public market.

30

Keeping Clean

Benjamin Franklin once said, "The secret of health is keeping clean inside and out." He laid down a great principle in these lines. He might have said, "The secret of physical, mental and spiritual health lies in keeping clean in body, mind and soul." The Lord has made provision for all three:

(1) For THE BODY—God has given elements (in soap) to cleanse THE BODY *without*, and CLEAN foods for *within*.

(2) For THE MIND—"Thy Word have I hid in mine heart [mind] that I might not sin against thee." "Wherewithal shall a young man cleanse His way? By taking heed thereto according to thy Word" (Psalm 119:11,9).

(3) AND SOUL—cleansing through the Redeemer's sin-atoning, sacrificial grace. "But he was wounded for our transgressions, he was bruised for our iniquities: the chastisement of our peace was upon him; and with his stripes we are healed" (Isaiah 53:5), ". . . for the transgression of my people was he stricken" (v.8) and "thou shalt make his soul an offering for sin" (v.10). "The blood of Jesus Christ, God's Son, cleanseth us from all sin" (I John 1:7).

Being made in the image of the so-called triune God, it is essential to our own welfare and happiness that we be clean in body, mind and soul (spirit).

Mind and Soul

One may be ever so meticulously clean in BODY, inside and out, but if he relishes and entertains filthy thoughts in the MIND, he is courting ailments, trouble, defeat and death. We may observe all the dietary laws, follow every physical health measure, but if we disregard the moral laws and the heart and mind are defiled, it is impossible for even the body to long remain well and strong. The immoral sins of the body (adultery, fornication, sex perversion, etc.) and of the mind (resentment, anger, jealousy, an unforgiving spirit) take a terrible toll upon a person's mind and body. We must be delivered from these things if we are to have the health and strength that the Almighty intended for us to enjoy. They must be eliminated as poisonous waste matter. Believer, our Saviour can make us "more than conquerors" over these destructive forces (Romans 6:23; 7:19–25; Philippians 4:8,9,13).

It is possible to take care of an automobile mechanically to the "Nth degree," by burning the best gasoline, having regular oil changes of top grade quality, regular grease jobs, giving every mechanical part and the electrical system the strictest care; yet if sand is put in the crankcase, the car, made to be a blessing, becomes a source of irritation and trouble. Similarly, this is what happens when doubt, unbelief, fear and evil thoughts are poured into the mind.

On the other hand, though you may take perfect care of every part of the car and *just neglect* changing or adding oil or changing the filter, you are headed for the commercial garage and big repair bills. Just so, we may observe the dietary law and every health measure faithfully, but if we neglect and disregard the moral and spiritual laws, the rules of life in God's Instruction Book, difficulty and grief are bound to overtake us.

Volumes could be written regarding the subject of the power

of the mind, its effect on and control over the body. Here, our spiritual relationship and fellowship with the Redeemer plays such an all-important part. The fact of negative impulses, being set up by man falsifying—lying—that is recorded on a "lie detector," is evidence that man's brain, nervous system and the entire universe are established on righteousness. Lying, deceit, hate, anger, jealousy, envy, suspicion, etc., cause the human mechanism, man's body, to revolt and register its disapproval. If this continues, it can finally bring about the breakdown of the entire body. These evil negative forces, as well as the positive, register every thought and expression in the body. (Although it is not accepted in our courts as absolute proof, yet the polygraph does register the various regular and irregular emotional and physiological impulses.)

Dr. N. Jerome Stowell, a well-known scientist, has testified in public lectures that he was an atheist until after his laboratory experiments measuring the wave lengths and power of thought in the human brain. In the case of a dying woman believer, as she praised God, the delicate needle of the scale moved positive as far as it could go. Then later the test was made on a man as he cursed God, and the needle went back to the negative side as far as it could. This is a sobering truth.

This is why Abraham Lincoln stated, "A man may not be responsible for the face he has at twenty, but he is responsible for the one he has at forty." Our inward electrical system does not only record on the face but on our kidneys, liver, heart, lungs, blood, and nerves. So let us keep in mind if we want to be well and strong, to constantly eliminate these unclean, destructive forces from our mind and heart by the grace of God made available to the nations and those whom He calls through Christ. (Read Matthew 11:27; John 15:3; Ephesians 5:26; I John 1:9; Colossians 3:5–10; II Timothy 2:21.)

The Body Within

The Lord has given several means of eliminating body wastes through the bowels, the kidneys, the lungs, and the skin. It is understandable that the more unclean, unnatural, artificial and foreign matter you take into the body the greater strain you place on these organs. If abuse continues over a period of years, the organs affected will finally rebel and break down. Doctors, hospitals, operations (and premature funerals) are then necessary. All sorts of artificial colorings and flavors, additives, preservatives, stimulants, with gluttonous amounts of devitalized sweets and fats, take their tremendous toll.

The first and most essential step toward the road to health is to keep these channels of elimination open. These wastes must be constantly cleansed from your body if you are to remain well. If you fail to change the oil in your car regularly, before long, sand, grit, metal shavings from your motor, as well as harmful acids created by combustion will destroy your motor. Likewise, wastes left in your body that are not eliminated will also do their insidious, destructive work.

The Bowels

The following story sounds almost incredible but I can vouch for it since I knew the couple well and of the incident firsthand.

The man's wife had to be committed to a mental institution because of her violence. An old country doctor knowing of the case said to her husband one day, "I have a firm conviction that your wife's trouble is caused by poisonous wastes being pent up in her body through lack of proper elimination. Faulty elimination of bowels and kidneys has not only pent up these poisons but has built up a pressure in her brain that is causing this irrational mental disturbance. I believe, if we can get her released from the institution long enough for treatment, she can be cured."

The arrangements were made with the institutional authorities for Mrs. D. to be released for this experiment. The treatment began with an old-fashioned enema which was repeated for a number of days. Other treatment included thorough cleansing of the entire intestinal tract, bowels, and kidneys. In a relatively short time my friend's wife was back to normal and was pronounced cured by the doctors of the institution. It was never necessary for her to return. This is just a small example of a miracle wrought by cleansing. Remember Benjamin Franklin's advice.

The best natural laxative is a daily helping of fresh fruit, eaten slowly. If your case is exceptionally stubborn have a helping of prunes or sip a glass of prune juice every morning; even a few figs work wonders. Walking a couple of miles a day, of course, is essential to anyone's health. (See Chapter 24.)

Parenthetically, may I inject: buy a good pair of shoes. Your feet are the foundation of your body, God's temple. Better own one good pair than several cheap ones, although it is good to have a pair for rotation. You'll never have another set of feet. Cheap, ill-fitting shoes can ruin them while good shoes will preserve them. If your feet 'go bad,' you cannot walk and the body is bound to deteriorate for lack of proper exercise. It is a good habit to remove your shoes a couple of hours before retiring and give your feet natural freedom and exercise which will help in relaxing you for the night. Use large comfortable slippers when possible. See that shoes are wide and long enough. Remember, every drop of blood must pass through your feet. And ill-fitting shoes can tension-you-up, tax your nerves and so affect your disposition.

And here is a special warning:

Beware of 'miracle' plastic sprays for shoes. The containers usually warn that even the vapor from them is harmful. Can you imagine what it would do to your lungs? Feet are also important. The Creator made leather to 'breathe.' When you seal shoe-leather with anything 'non-breathable' you, to that degree, jeopardize your health. It's still good sense to keep the feet dry in cold weather. But also take heed to the former suggestion unless you want "the hot-foot." In 1975–76 we were made more aware of the danger of aerosol sprays that effect the layer of ozone that encircles our planet.

Always, remember, "activate or disintegrate."

If you have a very severe case of constipation, may I suggest that you make yourself a cup of flaxseed tea each morning. Some take it raw—a small tablespoonful with a drink of water. It has a mild and healing action. Avoid harsh and strong laxatives.

One cause for constipation is the washing down of meals with drinks of various kinds. The water dilutes both the saliva and stomach gastric juices that the Lord made to break down and assimilate the food and which act as lubricants. The result? The body cannot carry on its regular digestive processes efficiently, and the food becomes lodged in the intestines, stomach and bowels, and develops toxins. All sorts of troubles are triggered off, beginning with gas pains to diseases that can take the life of the victim.

The Kidneys

Keep the kidneys cleansed with fresh clean water. If there is a question about your water supply, buy distilled water, which as a rule can be purchased at the food market. Keep out the phosphoric acids and dye coloring matter found in soft drinks, etc. I can't say it often enough: drink water and other fresh fruit juices between meals. Remember, if you insist on drinking with the meal, sip it. No drinks should be gulped.

The Skin

The skin is also an organ of elimination. It actually breathes. It is like a third kidney, because it eliminates as much urea as the kidneys. If the skin were painted or prevented from giving off heat, perspiration and waste, you would soon die from poisoning and overheating. Sweat glands throw off from one to twenty quarts of perspiration a day, depending, of course, on the temperature and activity. Perspiration also contains salt, potassium, iron, sulfuric, phosphoric and lactic acids. For this reason it is essential that you increase your salt intake during the summer months. If you perspire freely, suffer from the heat, headaches, etc., take salt tablets according to directions.

Lungs

Your lungs, also, are an organ of elimination. They take oxygen into the blood stream and are constantly expelling carbon dioxide and other waste gases from the body. Why should anyone overtax this delicately constructed mechanism by smoking and defiling it with nicotine, besides the number of other poisons found in cigarettes?

When various sicknesses and diseases come and the body breaks down, we have no right to say, "Why did God put this cancer, this tumor, or this affliction on me?" We bring them upon ourselves by improper care and a disregard for the laws of God. As believers, let us keep in mind that our bodies are the temples of the Holy Spirit of God, the habitation of God's own presence. We have been made custodians and stewards of them. Let us keep them clean and thereby well, to better praise and serve our all-wise and faithful Lord.

Note From the Author's Wife: For Women Only

I once discovered a lump on one of my breasts about the size of a pigeon egg. The natural reaction was to become panicky. Many of my friends had had trouble like this and their doctors usually recommended surgery. Sometimes this occurred over and over again to the same women. However, my husband soon calmed my fears, reminding me of the promises of God and the absolute, "For every effect there is a cause." We prayed and asked for wisdom to find the cause.

An incident out of the past flashed through my husband's mind: His father had almost died as the result of using a foot deodorant. It did stop the perspiration but also almost stopped his heart. It is as important that the skin breathe as the lungs. The skin also eliminates poisons as do the kidneys. When these poisons are blocked from excretion and remain in the body, plus absorbing foreign chemicals (such as "aluminum sulphate" which I found was in my deodorant), is it any wonder tumors and growths are formed?

My husband also suggested that I stop wearing the type of bra that hinders skin breathing, and wearing them too tightly can hinder the circulation of blood.

I changed deodorant—and sometimes simply used baking soda. I bought cloth bras that allowed circulation of air and did not wear them tightly. In seven to eight months this growth was reduced to the size of a small pea and disappeared within a year and never returned. I praise the Lord for giving us this knowledge, for without it my health might have been destroyed (Hosea 4:6). (I do not say, of course, that all such lumps are caused by these two things.)

31

The Masked Bandit

Psychosomatic Ills

Mayo Brothers of the famed Mayo Clinic of Rochester, Minnesota, reported a number of years ago that fifty percent of all hospital cases stem from mental causes, which have their roots in worry, fear and sorrow. They went on to state that if these victims had had a vital faith in God, they would never have had a physical breakdown. More recently the American Medical Association has raised the percentage even higher than this.

Dr. Charles E. Flowers, Jr., professor of obstetrics and gynecology of North Carolina University's School of Medicine, stated that "Sixty percent of all illnesses have psychological connotations." He declared that it must be recognized that emotional anxieties do contribute to ill health. We bring such difficulties upon ourselves, and yet they should not be found in 'the believer.'

Fear and Worry, Atheism

Dr. George W. Truett, the great Baptist pulpiteer from the South, preached a sermon in a sentence when he declared, "Worry is a mild form of atheism." Think it over. Doubt and unbelief are not only damaging but damning. It calls God a liar. When these insidious rebel forces move in, they clog up the entire being, as sand and grit thrown into a precision-made piece of equipment. Not only does the man fail to function properly but many times greater damage is done.

God created our body, brain and nervous system to operate on the principle of faith. What happens when we feed it on worry, fear and unbelief? The nervous system, like tiny little power lines, runs throughout your body alongside the blood vessels and tiny capillaries. *When FAITH* is in operation, you are relaxed and the entire system of heart, blood, nerves, and lungs carries on its wonderful healing and body-building processes. If for some reason sudden FEAR strikes you, the nerves, like tiny tentacles, clamp down on the blood vessels and cut off the flow of blood. If the shock of fear is strong enough, the blood is cut off almost completely from the brain and the person "faints." In other cases when fear's impact is not so severe but a feeling of "BEING AFRAID" grips you, then the blood's flow to the extremities of the body is hindered and the person actually does get "cold feet." *When you WORRY,* the result is not evident immediately but very subtle, for it creates a constant pressure on the nerves and therefore on the circulatory system of the whole body. The end result is more devastating because of this CONTINUAL nerve tension, which acts as thousands of road blocks in the arteries and capillaries, and hinders the normal rhythmic flow of blood from carrying on its healing processes.

Whenever and wherever the blood cannot flow normally to the various areas of the body, cells break down and die instead of being fed and built up. Sickness and disease follow and finally cell-breakdown is so great that the body is no longer able to function and the body collapses and death results. Worry actually kills!

Make God's Word "Dictator"

"I am the Lord thy God . . . Thou shalt have no other gods before me" (Exodus 20:2,3). God created your body, brain and nervous system to fear only One—that is, "the Lord thy God." When we fear anyone else or anything else, we become the author of the miseries that come upon us by our very disobedience to His command, "Fear not."

"The fear of man bringeth a snare" (Proverbs 29:25—Read Isaiah 51:12–16). How miserable are the people who *fear man,* public opinion, top religious leaders, opposing organizations, or even nations above God. What are these in the sight of our God? (Here read Isaiah chapter 40.) They are all like grass which shall be cut down. To God, the nations are like a "drop of a bucket, yea, they are as nothing before Him and less than nothing" (Isaiah 40:15–17).

The honor of men is as devastating as the fear of man. When we begin to pay undue honor unto men, soon we do not know which one to honor above the other. We then automatically begin to dishonor God, forgetting that all that man is, and has, comes from God. What do any of us have that we have not received (I Corinthians 4:6,7)? "How can ye believe which receive honor one of another and seek not the honor that cometh from God only?" (John 5:44).

Is it any wonder we have "split personalities" and so many nervous disorders, when we bow here, and do obedience there, and seek the favor of men rather than God? Paul reminds us that we should not give "eye service, as men pleasers, but as the servants of Christ doing the will of God from the heart" (Ephesians 6:6).

Make God your dictator. Settle it once and for all. Write it indelibly upon your soul that all others and all else shall be subordinate to Him and to His Word. You will never then be snared and robbed of all that is precious by "the masked bandit of fear and worry."

Divine Order

This, of course, takes into account God's order for the home. Making God your dictator means obeying His Word and commands. For husbands it means Christ-like love for their wives. For wives it means being subject to their husbands (Ephesians 5:21–23; I Peter 3:1–7). For children it means obedience to their parents (Ephesians 6:1–3). This is the secret of God's blessing and order in the home. In civil life it means being subject to "the higher powers [God's]. For there is no power but of God: the powers that be are ordained of God." (Read Romans 13:1–7.) In matters of spiritual authority God has given the order of the Church, and in general: "And we beseech you, brethren, to know them which labour among you, and are over you in the Lord, and admonish you; And to esteem them very highly in love for their work's sake" (I Thessalonians 5:12,13). Obedience to God's Word in all things is the key to all happiness. This will deliver from all fear and worry.

32

A Final Word

Pass It On

This book has been written with the hope of helping those who are sick and ailing and to keep others from suffering needlessly as I did for so long. I came near to being "destroyed for lack of knowledge." And may we never "reject knowledge" as many of God's people have done to their hurt and sorrow (Hosea 4:6,7). I have proved the truths of this book in my own body for over the past 40 years. I trust, reader friend, that you will pass it on to others that they may benefit and be delivered from the miseries that follow those who disregard God's Holy Law and Word. You may meet with rebuffs, ridicule and scoffing. If we are weak, these things will defeat us. If we are strong, it will spur us on the more to make the message of true deliverance known.

Stand Pat

"Life is a grindstone. Whether it grinds us down or polishes us up depends upon the stuff we are made of." Fear not; be of good courage; be not dismayed. God's Word, the history of God's people and experience are on our side. Let us keep up the good fight and we will win out to the inevitable victory of physical blessing, radiant health, and a happy mental outlook.

Hold your ground and stand fast in these truths. Remember, the Lord pays great dividends to the obedient; and recall, 'delays are not denials.'

Be Moderate

However, as important as these things are, yet I would not close this book without this word of caution: Let not the welfare of the body, which is the temple of God, eclipse the things of the Spirit. Let not nutrition, the building of the temple, take precedence over the Lord who dwells in it. Do not let diet and nutrition become an obsession so that it monopolizes your time and occupies the uppermost place in your thoughts. Let it rather be a *means* toward the *end* of blessing, that you may more fully glorify God in your spirit and in your body which are His.

Let us not forget we were sent into the world to make known the Redeemer, Who is the express image of the invisible God. He is all in all. May all these things be instrumental in exalting and extolling Him. He is our peace, our righteousness, and our life.

In the introduction, you will recall we saw that the number one interest of all people everywhere is health. Why is this? Because people love life, and without health there can be no real life. Sickness may be a living death, but still man will cling to any hope that life holds out. Man's greatest desire then, is LIFE, with the secret hope and longing for a perfect life; LIFE lived to the full; LIFE in complete satisfaction and contentment; LIFE, with every desire, benefit and good, fulfilled.

"All that a man hath will he give for his life," the devil said to God when he was seeking the Almighty's permission to attack Job (Job 2:4). Satan knew he spoke the truth and he would use man's chief desire to break his faith in God. There are such things as satanic attacks on the body today and we must recognize them and cast ourselves completely on our Lord for these deliverances. These attacks are temporary and will pass.

However, we must also recognize, because of man's transgression of God's law and the resultant curse, the body will ultimately wear out and decay (excepting Messiah's return). Take care of it as best we can, it will end up in a cemetery. But, this doesn't satisfy man. There is the innate desire within every man for life, LIFE—abundant and eternal, beyond the veil of death. This is what Messiah (Christ) came to bring. The Prophet Isaiah predicted concerning Him, "He was wounded for our transgressions . . ." and "He bare the sins of many." Read Isaiah 53. He restores and becomes the very tree of life from which man was driven because of his transgressions (Genesis 3). Life eternal dwells only in God, therefore, only God in Christ could declare, ". . . I am come that they might have life, and that they might have it more abundantly" (John 10:10). John wrote of Him, "All things were made by Him and without Him was not anything made that was made. In Him was life, and the life was the light of men" (John 1:3,4). This is the life that was purchased for us at the cost of the shed blood of God's lamb as given in type by Moses (Leviticus 1; 17:11). Do you enjoy this life?

This physical life can come to a close so abruptly. A bone caught in the throat, a virus, an auto or plane crash, and all this life is over. We can suddenly be cut off from this earthly existence a thousand ways. Therefore, the most important thing in all the universe is to have eternal life which alone dwells in God, and is manifested in Christ Jesus the Lord. "This is the record, that God hath given to us eternal life, and THIS LIFE IS IN HIS SON. He that hath the Son hath life, and he that hath not the Son of God hath not life" (I John 5:11,12).

Thank God, this life is a gift as was our physical life. This life also comes through seed—the seed of the Word of God. "Being born again, not of corruptible seed but of incorruptible, by the Word of God which liveth and abideth forever." When we receive this seed (the Word), then as Paul declares, "God sends forth the Spirit of His Son into our hearts crying, 'Abba, Father.'" This is what Jesus calls the new birth. We are then members of the new creation which can never pass away. When this old one falls in decay and corruption on the earth, we shall find ourselves in a new heaven and a new earth that shall never pass away. Reader, you too can enjoy this new and everlasting life set forth so simply in John 3:16, "For God so loved the world that He gave His only begotten Son that whosoever believeth in Him should not perish but have everlasting life." God's good news to the nations.

"Verily, verily, I say unto you, He that heareth my word, and believeth on him that sent me, hath everlasting life, and shall not come into condemnation; but is passed from death unto life" (John 5:24).

"That if thou shalt confess with thy mouth the Lord Jesus, and shalt believe in thine heart that God hath raised him from the dead, thou shalt be saved" (Romans 10:9).

The Abundant Life

King David knew the "over-flowing life" as he wrote, "My cup runneth over" (Psalm 23:5). We can also know this abundant life. It was this, Jesus offered as He stood in the Temple at Jerusalem at the feast of tabernacles, "and cried saying, *If any man thirst,* let him come unto Me, and drink. He that believeth on Me, as the Scripture hath said, out of his innermost being shall flow rivers of living water. (This spake He of the Spirit which they that believe on Him should receive: for the

Holy Spirit was not yet given, because that Jesus was not yet glorified)" (John 7:37–39).

Read very slowly, thoughtfully and repeatedly John chapters fourteen, fifteen and sixteen, asking the help of God's Spirit. The key to this *abundant* life is "If ye keep my commandments" (John 15:10). "These things have I spoken unto you that My joy might remain in you and that your joy might be full. This is My commandment that ye love one another as I have loved you" (John 15:11,12).

Sandwiched in between the Apostle Paul's great treatise on the miracle work of God's Spirit (I Corinthians 12 and 14) is the 'love chapter' (Ch. 13) which he calls "a more excellent way" in which he declares, *"Love never faileth"* (v.8). But this over-whelming love must be born of God's Spirit, not merely professed and 'man-made.' Paul likens the abundant life to one filled with wine when he wrote to Ephesus, "Be not drunk with wine wherein is excess but be filled with the Spirit" (Ephesians 5:18), and to Galatia "the fruit of the *Spirit* is *love, joy, peace.* . . ." (Galatians 5:22,23).

We are commanded then to be filled with His Spirit of love, joy and peace; therefore *we know it is His will.* On this premise we can claim just now immediately, this wonderful gift of His life-giving resurrection power. "And this is the confidence that we have in him, that, if we ask any thing *according to his will,* he heareth us: And if we know that he hear us, whatsoever we ask, *we know* that *we have* the petitions that we desired of him" (I John 5:14,15).

On the day of Pentecost there were two classes of people that witnessed this mighty out-pouring of God's Spirit on believers. *Some* sincerely asked, *"What meaneth this?"* And *others mocking* said, "These men are full of new wine" (Acts 2:12,13). But Peter said, *"This is that* which was spoken by the [Hebrew] Prophet Joel; And it shall come to pass in the last days, *saith*

God, I will pour out of my Spirit upon *all* flesh" (vs. 16,17). Not now only on prophets, kings and priests and the people of Israel, but upon *all* flesh as God in Christ through Israel reaches out to the whole world. "He is the propitiation [covering] for our sins; and not for ours only, but also for the sins of the whole world" (I John 2:2).

The Lord of Life

The Book of God begins with the Spirit of God breathing LIFE, light and order into being in the first temporal creation: and ends with His Spirit calling those who are under the curse of the old order of death, darkness and confusion, to partake of the new creation of peace, joy and *life eternal in the Redeemer.* "The Spirit and the bride say, Come. Let him that heareth say, Come. And let him that is athirst come. And whosoever will, let him take of the water of life freely" (Revelation 22:17). "I, Jesus, have sent mine angel to testify unto you these things . . . *I am the root and the offspring of David* and the bright and morning star" (v.16), "the *Lion of the tribe of Judah*" (Revelation 5:5) and the coming *"KING OF KINGS AND LORD OF LORDS"* (19:16).

In that day we shall know eternal HEALTH and the complete fulfillment of all HAPPINESS which shall never pass away and we shall sing the praises of our great God and Saviour throughout the endless ages of eternity. Amen.

A Closing Word

I must not close this 1976 edition of *God's Key to Health and Happiness* without a final word regarding a passage of Scripture which to me has become one of the most important in all the eternal Book of God. It was the first one (recorded) that Jesus quoted when He began His ministry. It is very fitting that it IS first, since food and eating is the number one desire of all men in every generation. And wrong eating is the cause of more trouble than anyone can dream or imagine.

Satan had just chided Jesus about his forty day fast with the scoffing challenge, "If thou be the Son of God command these stones to be made bread." (And having lived in Israel into our fifth year we are well aware of the abundance of stones in that Judean wilderness.)

Jesus countered with, "Man shall not live by bread alone." Unfortunately, when the translators read the next line they concluded that "by all that comes out of the mouth of God" meant only "every word that cometh out of the mouth of God," and so they put it down that way. However, there is more that comes out of the mouth of God than His Word and this is terribly important.

We read in Genesis 2:7 that, "God formed man out of the dust of the ground and breathed [out of His mouth] into his [man's] nostrils the breath of life." In Job 33:4 we read, "The Spirit of God hath made me and the breath of the Almighty hath given me life." This indicates that there is more that comes out of the mouth of God than His Word—It is the creative, life-giving breath of God, without which even the Word of God would be the deadness of the letter and as Paul writes, "the letter killeth but the Spirit giveth life."

God's two agents are His Word and His Spirit, both of which are absolutely essential in all that God has ever created or ever will accomplish. Knowing this, we should ask God to give us of His Spirit to understand His Word and that we might always be on the stretch, in search for the precious gold nuggets, the gems, the rubies and diamonds of His Truths as one who hunts for precious hidden treasure. Solomon reminds us that "all the things that thou canst desire" are not to be compared to this wisdom and full life, in which we find the right answers to all of our questions and His solutions to all of our problems.

Therefore, the *first* of every day we should partake to the full of the *"bread of LIFE,"* reading and obeying His life-magnetizing words; and drinking freely of the *"water of LIFE"*—His resurrection power, praying and praising without ceasing! We will then know the release from frustration and inferiority complexes that plague so many, and will be given the true success and prosperity He has promised for today and for all the days to come. This is *God's Key,* not only to health and happiness, but to *all* the blessings of heaven and earth, according to His riches in glory by the sin-atoning Redeemer (Joshua 1:8; Psalm 67:5,6; Isaiah 55:10,11; Jeremiah 15:16; Matthew 4:4; John 15:7–11; Philippians 4:19). Amen ('so be it established').